Dear Isabel and Dr. Weiss,

First, let me just say your assembly at our school was awesome. Listening to our students share their experiences about their breasts transported me back in time—I remember having so many of the same fears, and trying so hard to either hide the fact that I was wearing a bra with baggy sweatshirts or, at times, going through phases where I wanted to wear a thin white T-shirt so everyone knew! Talk about a confusing time . . . I also remember how my mom handed me a generic "growing up" book and was so embarrassed to talk about things. I definitely wish she had handed me your book, so I could have seen that there were so many other girls out there who were going through the exact same thing. This is an amazing project.

Jessica, high-school teacher

taking
care
of your
"GIRLS"

Also by Marisa C. Weiss, M.D.

7 Minutes

Living Beyond Breast Cancer

Marisa C. Weiss, M.D., and Isabel Friedman

Three Rivers Press
New York

A Breast Health

Guide for Girls, Teens, and In-Betweens

....

taking

care of

your

"GIRLS"

All information in this book is intended for your general knowledge only—and is not a substitute for medical advice or medical treatment. It is designed to support, not replace, regular care by a physician. Please consult your health-care professional on any question you may have. You should never disregard medical advice or delay in seeking medical advice because of something you read in this book.

Library of Congress Cataloging-in-Publication Data

Weiss, Marisa C.
  Taking care of your "girls" : a breast health guide for girls, teens, and in-betweens /
Marisa C. Weiss and Isabel Friedman.—1st ed.
    p. cm.
  Includes bibliographical references and index.
  1. Breast—Care and hygiene.   2. Teenage girls—Health and hygiene.   I. Friedman,
Isabel.   II. Title.
  RG493.W45 2008
  618.1'9—dc22   2008017457

ISBN 978-0-307-40696-5

Printed in the United States of America

DESIGN BY ELINA D. NUDELMAN

10 9 8 7 6 5 4 3 2 1

First Edition

Our book is dedicated to our close friend and champion,

Antoinette Passo Westphal

The embrace of your love, style, and compassion can be felt by girls and their families all around the world—now and for years and years to come.
Let every page in this book be one of your wonderful, sweet letters written to every girl who is growing up, becoming a woman, rising to the challenges, and feeling the power, joy, and comfort of her own strength.

Acknowledgments

We want to give heartfelt thank-yous to the rest of our family: Henry, Elias, and David.

Special thanks go to our other daughter-mother team, Lena Walker and Alice Weiss; our editor, Heather Jackson; and our literary agent, Linda Loewenthal, for their excellent guidance and dedication; and to Kathleen Mullaly, for her terrific art direction.

This book wouldn't have been possible without tremendous support from Hope Wohl, Cindy Pelton, Michele Zwiebel, Anne Altomare, Jennifer Paradis, Lisa Petkun, Patty and Gary Holloway, and the Breastcancer.org team and Board of Directors, and Beth Johnson, Bill Kennedy, David Felsen, and faculty from Friends' Central School; Elaine Thompson, Jack Lynch, Scott McKinnon, Robin Cohen, Al Denittis; Pat Nogar from Lankenau Hospital; Joan Countryman from Atlanta Girls' School; Elizabeth English from the Archer School for Girls; and David Midland and Sue McKenzie from the National Association of Health Education Centers.

We have deep appreciation for the tremendous support from the Westphal family: Ray Westphal, Amanda Radcliffe, Stevie Lucas, and Jeff Westphal. We are blessed by the Kelly Rooney Foundation and Save Second Base, and the dedication of Sean Rooney, Erin Dugery, and Kelly Day.

We are very grateful to school leaders Sr. Jean Levenstein, Dierdre Mecke, Steve Piltch, Helen Hamlet, and Judy Shea, and to the fabulous girls from Notre Dame Academy, Archbishop Prendergast, Lower Merion High School, Shipley, Merion Mercy Academy, Atlanta Girls' School, and the Coretta Scott King Leadership Academy, who shared their voices (their names were changed to protect their privacy).

Thanks for terrific support and guidance from Christine Pakkala, Ellen Weiss, Adele Friedman, Margo Weishar, Joanne Gilles-Donovan, Jamie and Marcy Margulies, Renee Dillon Johnson, Harley and Shari Foos, Nina Montee, Harvey Karp, Jessica Laufer, Stefania Magidson, Marge Tabankin, Joyce Ostin, Larry Nortor, Susanna Lachs, Lisa Glassner, Jaana Jovonen, Melanie Bone, Amy Davis, Alan Stolier, Judy Caper, Al Vernachio, Nancy Frandsen, Aileen Roberts, the 2006 Claniel Award, the John C. and Chara C. Haas Charitable Trust, and the Noreen Fraser Foundation.

Contents

INTRODUCTION: *Isabel's Take* 1

PART ONE *Knowing Your "Girls" Inside and Out*

1 *Breast Development: Hormones, Puffy Nipples,*
  Growing Breasts 9

2 *Breast Size and Shape: Just Right, Too Big,*
  Too Small, Uneven 27

3 *What's That? Noticing, Feeling, and Checking for*
  Breast Changes 43

4 *Skin Stuff: Stretch Marks, Breakouts, Rashes* 57

5 *Nipple Tips: Itches, Fluid, Hair, Inverted,*
  and Other Stuff 69

6 *Normal Breast Changes: Lumps, Cysts,*
  Thick Areas, Pain 79

PART TWO   *Taking Care of Your "Girls"*

7   Self-Image and Teasing: Standing Up for Yourself
    and Feeling Your Personal Power   95

8   Bras for You: Cami, Athletic, Underwire,
    Padded, Lace   117

9   Show Off, Cover Up, or Glide By? Dress to
    Express and Move with Confidence   137

10 When You Want Your Breast Size to Be Different:
    From Padded Bras to Surgery   151

11 From Tight Bras to Antiperspirants: Replacing
    Breast Cancer Fears with Facts   167

12 Think Pink, Live Green: A Planet-Friendly Guide
    for Healthy Breasts   193

Getting the Last Word   219

Resources   227

Index   233

taking
care
of your
"GIRLS"

Introduction
Isabel's Take

From Me to You

It's not easy to talk to anyone about the changes your body is going through—especially the private changes. You want to know everything but you don't want to feel uncomfortable learning about it. So how do you get answers to your questions? How do you find the reassurance that everything is going okay and figure out what to expect next? This can all happen in a bunch of ways. Someone in your family might take you aside for "a talk." You might learn some of the things at school or from friends. A book might show up in your room that has a lot of answers (like this one). Or maybe you'll see something in a magazine or on TV.

For me things were a little different. I grew up in a unique household. I'm not saying puberty wasn't a confusing time for me, because it was. But because both my parents are doctors (as are three of my grandparents), medical information has always been easy to get. I never had "the talk" because I heard talk about bodies all the time. I also have a very close and open relationship with my cousins and aunts on my mom's side of the family. Dinner conversations quickly get carried away, and we share lots of funny and embarrassing stories.

Years before my own breasts even started to develop, my mom and aunts would tell stories and pass down wisdom from their own experiences. Once my aunt Alice told my cousin Lena, eight, and me, ten, that when she was my age, she felt a bump in her breast. Worried that it might be breast cancer, Alice ran downstairs to tell her mother. Her mom—my grandmother—assured a panicked Alice that it was not breast cancer at all, but that her breast buds were starting to grow!

We all got a good laugh out of the story, but I had another feeling: huge relief! I'd had the same breast cancer scare with my breast bud as Aunt Alice did. That night, Lena and I stayed up late and talked and she said she had been scared too. Even two girls from a family of doctors could freak out about these big changes! From that point on, I knew how important it was to learn about what was going on with my own body; I did not want to be scared every time I noticed a change.

By the time I was eleven years old, I had read through books and talked to friends and family. But I was still not entirely satisfied with the information. My mother is a breast cancer doctor, so I figured that she mainly knew what could go *wrong* with breasts. My father is a pediatrician, but I wasn't going to ask him *anything* about my breasts. Lena, at nine, had not yet started puberty, although she was just as curious about all the changes that I was going through. I also wanted to be prepared to teach Lena when she would go through puberty herself. Our joint fascination and eagerness to learn led us to create "nipple books." These were books we kept that helped us explore and understand what was going on with our bodies.

That summer, I began to notice more and more how different women's breasts were from each other and from mine. There were so many different shapes and sizes! I was already used to looking at human bodies in a scientific way because of my doctor parents, and this was like my own little observational study. On the beach and around town, Lena and I would observe the different kinds of breasts we saw, then come home and draw them in our nipple books. It was a fun way to spend time together and also to learn about our bodies.

You can see some of my illustrations here, and a bunch more at

TakingCareOfYourGirls.com. Most of my illustrations were realistic, others more imaginative, but in recording the "findings" of our "study," we came to one conclusion: every set of breasts is different and unique. It took me a while to realize that everything I had read about breasts and breast development applied to breasts that looked completely different. Lena and I thought that was pretty cool.

Then another question came to mind: how can you know you're normal when every girl and woman around you have breasts that look different from yours?

I learned then, and have come to realize even more now, that every girl experiences confusion and shared fears about her body as she grows up. Creating our nipple books helped Lena and me relieve those fears and make the best of all of the changes. Turning our worries into laughs allowed us to enjoy those exciting times in our lives. We weren't making fun of these different kinds of nipples and breasts; we were just being honest that the differences were there. Not everyone was going to look the same, and that was just fine.

It was five years later that I showed my nipple book to my mom. She thought it was great, and that just reinforced for me that my and Lena's curiosity was normal. Mom was pleased and surprised that we had taken notice of all the natural differences among women.

Now that I'm seventeen, I flip through my nipple book and giggle at some of the silly drawings I made, but I also appreciate how useful it was for me growing up. I know that not every girl is able to ask questions, express her concerns, or share her fears as easily as Lena and I did. Having this kind of relationship was so important to me—and would have a big positive influence on any girl.

And that's why I'm here for *you*. During puberty, your body can change faster than you can keep up with it, and it's not easy to find the answers to all the questions you have. This book draws upon my experiences and my mom's medical knowledge, and will help resolve your concerns and put your fears about breasts (your "girls") to rest with fun, easy-to-understand, reliable, meaningful information. Peppered throughout the book are tidbits of my perspective, for a girl-to-girl

from the "nipple book" of Isabel Friedman, age 11

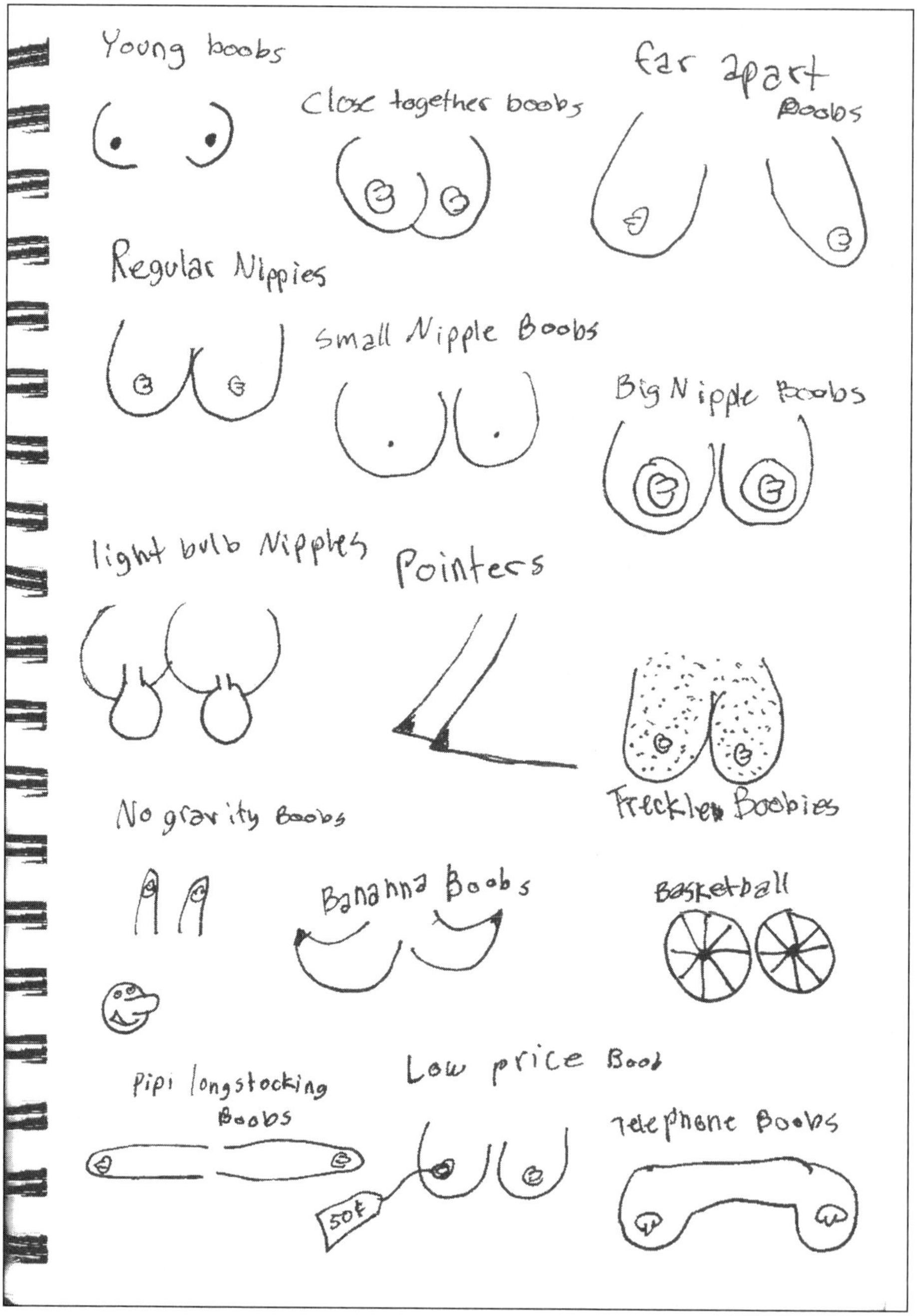

view, plus tons of other girls' stories, on all the subjects we cover. You're probably full of ideas and stories too. Please share them with me and other girls at our Web site, TakingCareOfYourGirls.com. Helping each other makes us all feel strong, smart, taken care of, and comforted. It feels much better knowing that we're all in this together.

We hope you find our book helpful and enjoyable!

Isabel Friedman

Mom to Mom: A Word from the Weiss

The goal of our book, *Taking Care of Your "Girls,"* is to take care of *our* girls by addressing their fears, questions, attitudes, and concerns about breast development and breast health. The information in this book is meant to empower them to become smart, healthy women with strength, confidence, and spirit.

Complete breast development, from the very start to the final finish, occurs over ten years. Growing breast tissue is more sensitive than full-grown breasts—since the food, water, beverages, and air our daughters take in become the building blocks for her new breast tissue, forming the foundation of her future breast health.

There is growing evidence that today's young girls have little knowledge about breast health, and this affects their physical and emotional well-being. From underserved young girls with limited access to health care and health/wellness information to the most educated and privileged girls in private schools, lack of information and misinformation about what it means to have healthy breasts are pervasive among girls today.

Our nonprofit organization, Breastcancer.org, together with the Lankenau Hospital, recently surveyed more than three thousand Philadelphia-area public and private school girls in the sixth through twelfth grades. The results were shocking:

- Although many girls are interested in hearing about breast health from their doctors, they often encounter different doctors with each visit and are unable to build a rapport enabling them to ask personal questions.

- About 90 percent of mothers say they'd like to talk to their daughters about breast health, but only about 30 percent have had the conversation.

- Over 30 percent of girls have perceived a normal change in their breasts to be a sign of breast cancer.

- More than 20 percent of girls think breast cancer is caused in part by infection, tanning, drug use, stress, breast injury, or bruising; however, none of these is a risk factor.

- Few girls know how to keep their breasts healthy.

The way in which girls and young women feel about themselves has a direct impact on the way they perceive themselves in every aspect of their lives. Self-confidence and self-esteem especially empower young girls to take on the challenges of life and reach their fullest and greatest potential.

It's us—their moms or other key trusted people in their lives— whom our girls want to be their source of this essential information about breast health. So it's up to us to get the conversation started in an age-appropriate, sensitive, responsive, respectful, and accessible way. Plus we have to keep our ears and eyes wide open and tuned in to their circles of influence: the people they look up to, the images they aspire to, their media sources, and the always-changing technologies they use to plug into the outside world.

Your love and dedication, supported by the information in *Taking Care of Your "Girls,"* can make a life-enhancing and life-saving difference in the lives of our girls today and better serve the health of our future generations.

Marisa C. Weiss, Mom and M.D.

part one

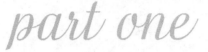

knowing your "girls" inside and out

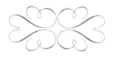

My breasts are very small. When my friends make comments about them, I tell 'em: "They're coming! They're just on back order."

Quinn, 15

Breast Development:

Hormones, Puffy Nipples, Growing Breasts

There were times I would pray to God, "I will do anything you like, I will do everything my parents say, but I do *not* want boobs!" It was awful starting to develop. You don't know what's going to happen next. And I just wanted to return back to the life I knew without all these problems.

Kelly, 13

I would rather talk to my older sister about my breast development than my parents. She doesn't ask me five hundred follow-up questions.

Sara, 12

I can tell you, every night—even when I was 11, and my girlfriends were kind of starting to get their period then, starting to develop something, I can remember—I was raised Catholic—I would pray: "Our Father, God bless Mommy, Dad, Mickey, Chrissie, Casey, Kansas"—who was my brother's dog—"and please God, let me wake up tomorrow with some boobs." That was the prayer. I can tell you exactly what it was because I spent years saying it.

Lizzie, 18

I knew a lot more about growing breasts than other people. And I was talking with a friend when a mother who was listening in asked, "How do you know all this?" I guess because I grew up the baby in my family, so I was learning about breast development and breast cancer from everybody older than me.

Mary Jane, 14

Well, all my friends think they will never have breasts. And it's not funny—because a lot of girls feel this way.

Sara, 13

I wished we had the talk about breast development *before* it occurred, not when the breasts first started to appear. We had the menstrual talk, but somehow breasts were left out.

Elena, 12

At my aunt's house, I pulled my mom aside to privately tell her that my boobs all of a sudden had started hurting. She said, "Ohhhh, you're growing breasts," and then she turned around and told my aunt everything I had just said.

Alexandra, 11

Girls in my school must get changed in the main room for gym class. At first some girls tried to sneak off and change in the bathroom, but the teachers caught them and made them change with everyone else. Now we're all used to it. We have no choice.

Susanna, 12

I started developing before everybody else. Between fifth and sixth grade I grew boobs and grew about six inches taller. It was ridiculous: I was so out of proportion.

Sasha, 18

Breast Development

When I was seven, I liked the whole idea of having boobs because everybody had them. Me and my friends would try on my mom's bra and laugh about it. We didn't really understand. I guess I thought that one day I'd just wake up and everything would be different. Only later did I realize how awkward the growing-up part would be.

Lena, 14

When I first got breasts, no one knew because I wore so many layers. A big T-shirt *and* a sweatshirt were the perfect solution. I was against even owning a bra. I wouldn't talk about it with my mom or anybody— and when the words came up I just pretended not to hear. My friends and I pretended we were disgusted by the whole idea of a bra, even though secretly we knew we needed one.

Emily, 15

Later, when I started high school, I was thinking that it's a lot more normal to have breasts there and I wanted to fit in and have fun—so I should just embrace it. But even so, I am still uncomfortable with them.

Megan, 17

The first things that changed about my body when my breasts started to grow were my nipples. They got so puffy I had to wear a tight camisole under my clothes to flatten them down.

Katie, 16

When my breasts began growing, they started showing through my shirts. I went through great lengths to hide them. I'd even use tape.

Lena, 14

[Breasts can even be an issue for boys, as this quote shows!] Our basket-ball team needed to practice some drills, so the coach divided our team in half: shirts versus skins. I was praying that I would be on the shirt team so no one would tease me about my, um, breasts. But no, of course that didn't happen. The coach put me on the skins team and ordered me to take off my shirt—but I pretended not to hear. Then he started yelling at me, "Take off your shirt!" I was horrified—completely embarrassed from my head down to my toes. Still I kept my shirt on. There was *no way* I was going to take off my shirt.

Ben, 16

First Things First

You know how when you're driving down the highway things pass by so fast, it can all look like a blur? Well, that's what breast development can feel like if you are a fast bloomer. And have you ever been stuck on the side of the road while other cars whiz by you? That's what growing breasts can feel like if you're developing slowly. Plus there are a lot of feelings rolled in: excitement, frustration, curiosity, embarrassment, discomfort, fun, confusion, fear, and hope.

Knowing what to expect will make you feel better and less uncertain. Knowledge really is power. This chapter will give you a "road map" that will help you understand and keep track of your own unique breast development.

Here's the Scoop

Breast development requires many steps and takes a bunch of twists and turns, starting inside your mom's uterus, making the greatest progress during puberty, then adding the finishing touches after high school. Let's tackle each step along the way.

In Your Mom's Uterus

Breast growth starts when you are barely three weeks—when you're just a tiny ball of cells called an embryo. Two little ridges of special tissue, called *mammary ridges,* form on top of your skin between your armpits and your thighs.

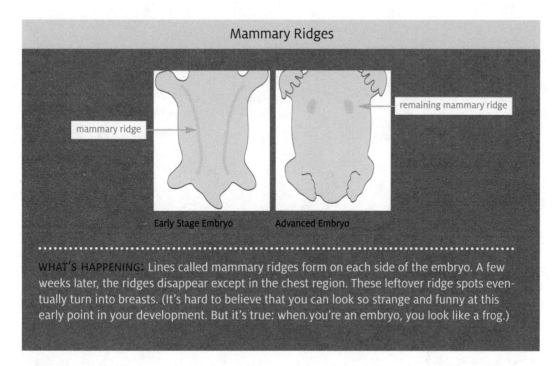

Mammary Ridges

mammary ridge

remaining mammary ridge

Early Stage Embryo   Advanced Embryo

WHAT'S HAPPENING: Lines called mammary ridges form on each side of the embryo. A few weeks later, the ridges disappear except in the chest region. These leftover ridge spots eventually turn into breasts. (It's hard to believe that you can look so strange and funny at this early point in your development. But it's true: when you're an embryo, you look like a frog.)

The ridges look like two stretched-out letter Cs, lying back to back. Weeks later, they all but disappear except for a small area on each side of your chest. Then, over the last six months of pregnancy, the leftover mammary ridge cells get to work making the very beginnings of your breasts.

First mammary ridge cells build up on top of the skin to form the nipples and the areolas. A nipple is the peak in the center of your breast, while the areola is the round, somewhat darker bumpy skin around the base of the nipple. A small pit or dent forms in the middle of the nipple, like the hole in the middle of a volcano. (Milk comes out of this opening during breast-feeding, sort of like a sprinkler or shower head.)

While nipple "construction" is under way, other mammary ridge cells dip beneath the surface to create the *breast bud*—the smallest and simplest version of the breast gland (milk-making "factory"). Little shoots sprout off the bud like little fingers on a hand. These fingers are

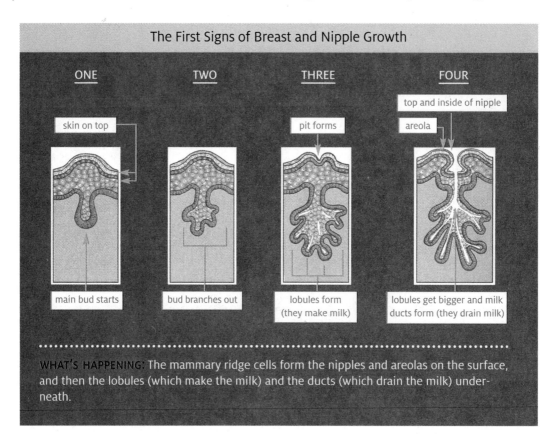

The First Signs of Breast and Nipple Growth

ONE — TWO — THREE — FOUR

top and inside of nipple

skin on top   pit forms   areola

main bud starts   bud branches out   lobules form (they make milk)   lobules get bigger and milk ducts form (they drain milk)

WHAT'S HAPPENING: The mammary ridge cells form the nipples and areolas on the surface, and then the lobules (which make the milk) and the ducts (which drain the milk) underneath.

the *lobules*, made up of milk-making cells. Next, pipes called *ducts* form between the lobules and the nipple. The ducts are responsible for draining the milk out to the opening in the middle of the nipple. At this stage of the game, the whole breast bud is tiny and too small to feel.

Breast Break

Breast development takes a break between the day you're born and the start of puberty. Your body has tons of other important work to do as you grow from a little baby into a young girl. It needs this "breast break" in order to grow taller and wider and to develop all of your other body parts.

Puberty

Sooner or later puberty rolls in—the time when your body changes from a girl's into a young woman's. A rise in the female hormones estrogen and progesterone gets the whole breast development show restarted. These hormones, made in your ovaries, travel to your breasts, delivering the message to get back to work.

The restarting of breast development is usually the first sign of puberty and the completion of your breast growth marks the end of puberty. All the other changes, like growing pubic hair, getting your period, getting taller, and having your hips get wider, happen in between.

The Breast Bud Forms a Lump

First, the breast bud behind each nipple gets bigger. It can feel like a little stone, pebble, blueberry, or grape. And it can be sensitive, tender, and sometimes painful.

The breast bud can appear in one breast for weeks or months before the bud on the other side starts to grow. One breast bud may be bigger than the other. They might blossom into breasts right away or hang around for a while before they go on to form breasts.

girl to girl

I think of the "breast break" period as the calm before the storm. Everyone your age looks the same, boys and girls, so all emotions surrounding development are non-issues. Sometimes I think, *Wouldn't it be nice if we were all just little kids again and totally carefree?* Yeah, it would be nice to a certain extent, but then you'd miss out on all the fun and exciting parts of getting older.

girl to girl

I was so proud of my breasts when they first started coming in. All the women around me had breasts, and now I was growing my own set! My breast development was a sign that I wasn't a little girl anymore, and I was very excited about that.

It's very common for girls to worry about breast cancer when they feel a new lump that doesn't go away—particularly when it's only on one side. But all of these changes are normal. There's no need to worry (Chapter 11 will give you a lot more information about this).

The Nipples and Areolas Get Going

Right after the breast buds start growing, the nipples and areolas get puffy, bigger, and darker. They can also feel itchy, painful, and more sensitive to the touch.

While the breast bud can't be seen, the puffy nipple/areola combination can look like a big mosquito bite and show through your clothes. Puffy nipples or areolas are often the first sign of breast development

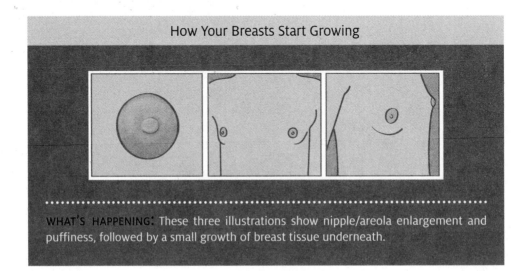

How Your Breasts Start Growing

WHAT'S HAPPENING: These three illustrations show nipple/areola enlargement and puffiness, followed by a small growth of breast tissue underneath.

isabel and her cousin lena's take

Lena: When my breasts began growing, they started showing through my shirts. I went to great lengths to hide them. I'd even use tape.

Isabel: I remember I did that once. During the summer, one day when I just did not feel like wearing a bra, and I was developed enough that I still had the mosquito bite nipple thing—and they were very visible. I either didn't have a bra that I could wear or I just didn't want to, so I taped my nipples down. I wanted to wear a shirt without a bra and without my nipples showing.

Lena: Yes, it was really hard during the summer to hide them because everybody was wearing these tiny shirts and all. So what I did was wear my bathing suit as much as possible—even though I rarely went swimming—because it worked as a bra. It would be the hottest day, and I would be wearing it and then this long shirt. I would be dying of heat. But I just did it anyway.

Isabel: Why?

Lena: So that nobody could see them.

that other people can see—making you feel very self-conscious—even before there is any breast tissue growth underneath.

Breast Gland Tissue Starts Growing

After your nipples and areolas get bigger, the breast buds underneath blossom further into the breast glands—the part that makes and drains milk.

The lobules and the milk ducts start up where they left off when you were born, branching again and again, like a tree in full bloom or a hand with many fingers. As this process

girl to girl

The puffy nipple thing stinks even more because the kinds of training bras available for girls are bad! A lot of the thin cotton training bras don't do squat to help conceal puffy nipples. I still see middle school girls who wear bad bras and you can clearly see the outline of their nipples. I fell victim to "nipple-itis" a few times when I was developing, too, and it's not fun.

How Your Breasts Continue to Grow

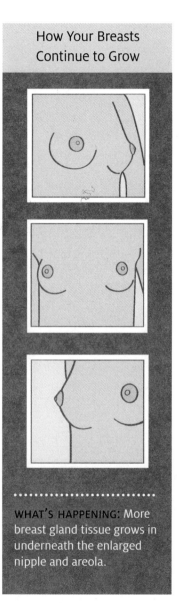

progresses, the breast tissue gets bigger and thicker. Fat fills in around the lobules and ducts and provides a protective cushion for these delicate and sensitive structures.

The breasts grow straight out before they grow from side to side. That's why they may look cone-shaped and pointy in the beginning. But over time they will get rounder and fuller.

While the nipples and areolas stay puffy, they can look like a little hill on top of a big mountain (breast tissue). Eventually the areolas flatten and the nipples in the middle get bigger and stick out more.

Later, the nipples and areolas stay about the same size while the breast underneath continues to get larger and rounder.

Some girls have nipples that point inward like a belly button that goes in (an "innie") rather than one that sticks out (an "outie"). Even though there is a medical term for this—*inverted nipples*—it's totally normal. (Chapter 5 has more information on all kinds of nipple variations.)

Nipple and areola size and color vary a lot from girl to girl; no two nipple-areola sets are the same. Big breasts with a small nipple-areola set, small breasts with a big set, or medium breasts with "mixed doubles" (large areolas and small nipples) are all completely normal. Nipples and areolas also come in different colors: light or dark shades of pink, beige, purple, brown, and black. A mixture of these colors might blend into one shade, or these colors may be pieced together like a mosaic or a patchwork quilt. You can also get freckles or other kinds of skin spots on your nipples and areolas. And sometimes the nipples are a slightly different color than your areolas.

Finishing Touches: These Breast Changes Are Going to Take Some Time

On average, it takes four years for girls to complete most of their breast growth. Sometimes it happens faster—over a few years—and sometimes it happens slower, such as over eight years.

Breast growth is not always continuous. Don't be surprised or worried if your breasts start growing, stop, start again, stop, and then finish. Plus the speed of your breast growth can change: sometimes fast, sometimes slow. One side might grow faster than the other side.

Over time, your breasts will get rounder just like the rest of your body, including your hips and rear end. Breasts reach their full size and shape by the time you're twenty-five, so you can't be sure that your breasts are full-grown until then. But it's really not until pregnancy that your breasts completely mature and learn how to make and drain milk for breast-feeding.

When Your Breasts Finish Growing

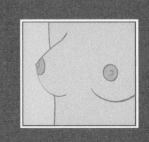

WHAT'S HAPPENING: As your breasts finish growing, the areolas flatten to the level of the breast and the nipples continue to stick out. The breast shape is full from front to back and side to side.

Any Questions?

Why do some boys get breasts?

You may have noticed that some boys grow breasts too. The medical term for enlarged breasts in males is *gynecomastia*—which means "woman-like breasts." Another not-so-polite word you might have heard to describe a boy's breasts is *moobs* (short for "man boobs").

girl to girl

I tried to help my cousin feel more confident about her changing body by being confident myself. I was always open about the subject and never tried to make her feel uncomfortable. I thought that if it looked like I had no insecurities, it would be easier for her to move past her own. But the truth was, I was self-conscious about my breasts—just in a different way than she was.

Believe it or not, most boys (about two-thirds) get some breast enlargement during puberty. Boys may even grow breasts earlier and bigger than girls their own age. Usually this breast growth goes away within a few years.

Really big boy breasts that look like a woman's breasts are uncommon. But either way, it's a very embarrassing problem, particularly during the summer when boys are expected to go shirtless at the beach.

I noticed my friend Jack has breasts. Why? And how should I deal with it?

As funny-looking as boy breasts might appear, you have to stop yourself from making fun of someone in this situation. The hurt feelings can go deep down and leave emotional scars that can last many years. Take a second to put yourself in his shoes; you wouldn't want to be made fun of.

Being overweight is often the most common cause of breast enlargement in boys. Hormones are another common cause—these are special protein "messengers" in the blood that tell the breasts to grow. The much higher level of female hormones and the much lower levels of male hormones in girls are the main reasons why girls grow breasts and boys usually don't.

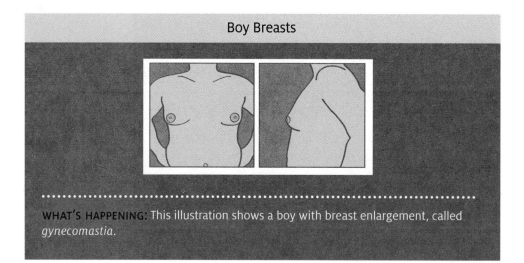

Boy Breasts

WHAT'S HAPPENING: This illustration shows a boy with breast enlargement, called *gynecomastia.*

Breast Development

Everyone has a balance of both boy and girl hormones. In boys, there are more boy hormones than girl hormones. In girls, there are more girl hormones than boy hormones. In some boys, the girl hormones cause breasts to form. In some girls, the boy hormones can limit breast growth. Over the years, as the balance of hormones changes, breast growth can also change.

Certain products contain substances that can act like hormones. For example, lavender oil and tea tree oils have been associated with breast enlargement in boys before puberty (these oils are present in some soaps, moisturizers, shampoos, and hair care products).

Some boys are born with an inherited genetic condition that can result in enlarged breasts.

Certain medicines can make breasts bigger—but most of these medicines are taken by adult men (not boys). About half of adult men develop breast enlargement over time. All the things that make breasts bigger in boys can also happen to men. Drinking too much alcohol is another cause in men.

Men who feel very self-conscious about the appearance of their breasts can go to a doctor (a plastic surgeon) to have them made smaller. Afterward the area can be reshaped so it looks normal. In fact, breast reductions are one-third as common in boys 18 and younger as breast enlargements for girls from the same age group. (In 2007, there were 2,758 breast reductions performed on boys and 7,882 breast enlargements done on girls.)

Why do some girls' "girls" grow faster than others?
Rate of breast growth depends on all kinds of things—just like growth spurts as you get taller. But what's very different about breast growth is that your breasts can keep on growing, filling out, and changing throughout your life, whereas your final height stays the same over the long run (at least until you're a much, much older person, when you can shrink ☹). The three biggest factors that determine rate of breast growth are the hormone levels in your body, your weight, and the pattern of growth in your family. Your age matters

less. So if you're an A cup at 14, you might still develop C-cup "girls" by age 20.

Why are my breasts so tender?

It's very common for newly growing breasts to be painful. You may have tingling, tenderness, shooting pain, extra sensitivity, itching, crawling sensations, or sharp or dull aches. Breasts are very delicate, sensitive parts of your body, especially when they first start growing.

These various feelings may come on without any notice. Or they may be brought on by touching, light pressure from your clothes, lying on your stomach, hugs, changes in position, or physical activity such as sports and exercise. These uncomfortable feelings usually get much better when your breast development is over. Breast pain that comes before your menstrual period and other kinds of breast discomfort will be discussed in Chapter 6.

Is there a normal nipple and areola color?

Your nipple and areola are usually darker in color than the skin on the rest of your breast, but sometimes their color is the same and occasionally it may be lighter. The color difference can range from slightly darker to much darker, and as you mature, the color tends to get even darker.

girl to girl

The first time I noticed nipple color variation was with our live-in babysitter. She was trying on clothes in front of me when I got a glimpse of her breasts. The color of her nipples was so close to the color of her skin that for a second I thought she didn't have nipples at all! I was only 9 years old at the time and it fascinated me.

Why is the skin of the nipple and areola a different texture than the rest of my breast?

The areola's thick skin provides extra protection from bumps and scratches since this part of your breast sticks out beyond most other parts of your body. This special skin also acts as a shield for all of the sensitive nerve endings underneath it and helps protect against a baby's saliva and strong sucking action during breast-feeding.

The little bumps on the areolas are called Montgomery glands (see diagram below). They make a very small amount of mucus, which you usually don't see, to help keep your nipples and areolas nice and soft (especially later on, during breast-feeding). Don't squeeze these bumps because scar tissue can form.

Why do newborn babies have breasts?

Most newborn girls and boys have a small amount of breast enlargement from exposure to their mom's high hormone levels during pregnancy. But these baby breasts usually go away within the first few weeks after birth.

How can my mom (or someone else close to me) bring up these subjects with me?

When we got this question we decided to toss it right back to girls like you. After all, you're the experts! If you could, what advice would you give your parent about how to start talking to you? Here's what girls like you told us:

- I would hope they would say, "I know you're going through a lot of changes with your body, and you are not the first girl to go through this. If you have any concerns, I would be more than happy to talk with you about anything you need or want to know about keeping healthy."

- I think they should ask me how I feel about developing breasts, and does it make me feel upset or strange? I would like them to bring it up slowly and to sound understanding—and to share their own experiences with me.

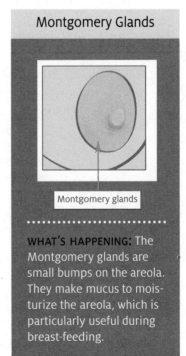

Montgomery Glands

Montgomery glands

WHAT'S HAPPENING: The Montgomery glands are small bumps on the areola. They make mucus to moisturize the areola, which is particularly useful during breast-feeding.

- "Sooo . . . booooooobs . . . let's talk!"

- I would probably want my *sister* to tell me about some of her experiences while she was going through her developmental process. I'd also like to hear about any possible problems or abnormalities I should be looking out for.

- "I want you to be healthy and safe . . . so we need to talk about breast problems that are possible for you, and how we can prevent them."

- Maybe she could say, "I know it may not be the most important thing on your mind, but this is a subject that can have a drastic effect on your self-esteem and be important to your physical health."

- "Well, honey, how are the 'ladies' doing? They good? Awesome!"

- "How are you feeling about your body?"

- I don't know that it's a specific choice of words, more that they have to approach the situation with a casual attitude. If they prepared carefully exactly what they would say, it would probably be awkward.

- "I just want to inform you of some of the potential risks with your breasts. It is important to have enough information to respond intelligently if a problem were to arise."

- "I know this might be awkward, but . . . Don't worry, everyone has questions about it! And you can talk to me whenever!"

- I really wouldn't care how it was brought up. I would rather it be brought up by a female close relative or close female family friend.

- I wouldn't mind my mom bringing it up and I would be fine with however she decided to approach it, because we are very close.

- "Just so you know, we should talk about the things that most schools don't cover. No one really talks about how to keep your breasts healthy, so I am going to tell you what I know. . . ."

- They could say anything to me. It's just a conversation starter to many topics, and this topic of breast cancer is very important with the constant advances and confusion of cancer itself.

- They should bring up a person we all know of that has breast cancer, what they did about it, how it could be prevented, et cetera.

- Just start talking.

All of the above advice from girls just like you can apply to any caregiver or trusted person. Feel free to apply that advice to an aunt, a grandma, a best friend, or whomever you feel comfortable talking to.

You can share your stories at TakingCareOfYourGirls.com.

I wear a semi-padded bra to look good in clothes, but when I go swimming at my pool I feel there isn't enough there to fill in a bathing suit top. What should I do?

Janelle, 18

2

Breast Size and Shape:

Just Right, Too Big, Too Small, Uneven

I am smart and have a lot of friends, but I've never felt pretty because my breasts are so small. I'm barely an A and I've been 5'10½" since tenth grade.

Lori, 18

I've been in beauty pageants, and breast size matters. They use tape to lift them up, but on me there are no breasts to even tape up or move together.

Tanya, 17

My cousin is petite like her mom, but she has broad shoulders like her dad, and surprise: she has really big breasts like her dad's mom! I am always amazed when I see her, especially next to her small-breasted mother. In contrast, I have my mother's body from the waist up, but my legs and rear end are just like my dad's. Go figure!

Ellen, 17

In biology class in sixth grade I remember telling the class that genes don't always matter with breast size because, example A, my mom is very voluptuous . . . and then I continued to announce to the whole class while pointing at my chest: "But see? I'm flat as a pancake!"

Ella, 14

My sister always told me how small I looked and how she had much bigger and better breasts. Well, now that she's lost weight and I've matured more, it seems that karma is playing its role. Now she's a 34A and I'm a 34B!

Melissa, 16

I was the last one in my class to start growing breasts and the last one to finish. By the very end of high school, I was bigger than all of my friends.

Meredith, 19

When I was starting to develop, one breast was way smaller than the other, but eventually they evened out to a regular size.

Susan, 18

My friend always gets teased about having tiny breasts, so she decided to stuff her bra with my mother's jelly breasts. Then once when she was doing a fancy trick, one of them flew out. She was so embarrassed!

Ping, 15

First Things First

Breast size grabs more attention than any other breast topic. And it's no surprise—our breasts are the most visible signs of puberty, and they seem to change almost every day. Plus there are pictures of breasts everywhere. They're staring right at you on nearly every television show and magazine page. Celebrities' breasts spill out of their clothes, and extreme-makeover shows make big ones even bigger. It's just about impossible *not* to compare your breasts to everyone else's. Between the

Breast Size and Shape

big breasts on the swimsuit model and the perky ones on the teenage rock star, you might feel you just don't measure up. With all of this going on, you can forget your own strengths and feel not so good about yourself.

This chapter will give you all the information you need about the size and shape of your "girls," so you can know what to expect, have less anxiety and disappointment, and feel better about yourself and your body. Of course, learning how to enjoy being *you* takes a while—but it's all really worth it. Why? Because your life is a gift: there *is* only one you!

Here's the Scoop

One size never fits all. There is no "perfect," "right," or "normal" breast size. Each girl has her own special look, size, shape, and proportion—thank goodness—because life would be really boring if everyone were the same.

A Matching Pair—or Not

The size and shape of both breasts can match, or one side can be bigger than the other.

Breast size depends on a bunch of different things: genes, nutrition, body type, age, and hormones. Few of these factors work alone; most of them depend upon each other.

Family Genes and Breast Size

The genes you inherited from your mother and father have the biggest influence on the size of your

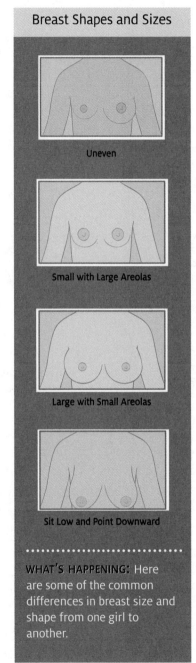

Breast Shapes and Sizes

Uneven

Small with Large Areolas

Large with Small Areolas

Sit Low and Point Downward

WHAT'S HAPPENING: Here are some of the common differences in breast size and shape from one girl to another.

breasts. Genes act like an instruction manual—they control your body's function from day to day, week to week, and year to year. They tell your breast tissue when to start developing, how fast to grow, what shape and size to take on, and when to stop growing. You were born with your own set of unique genes, which can't be changed. Big-breast genes can't be turned into small-breast genes, and small-breast genes can't be made big—and that's okay. Every girl has her own combination of genes that make her breasts and development unique. But your genes don't act alone. They work closely with your hormones, weight, and a lot of other factors.

Nutrition, Weight, and Breast Size

You've probably heard the saying "You are what you eat." Well, it's true: the foods you eat can directly affect the health of your breasts. Food can also sometimes affect the *size* of your breasts.

In general, the different food elements—carbohydrates, protein, and fats—have a similar effect on breast size. One type of food can't make your breasts bigger or smaller. But regularly consuming foods that contain hormones, like some non-organic dairy products over an extended period of time, could cause an unhealthy increase in breast size. Also, eating a lot of high-calorie processed foods results in a rapid rise in blood sugar, which in turn triggers high insulin levels. Insulin is the hormone that tells your body to store the extra energy as fat; it can also stimulate unhealthy extra cell growth. Weight and body fat have a big influence on breast size. In fact, the biggest difference between small and large breasts is the amount of fat they contain. Of course, you can be of slender build and have large breasts, and you can have a larger build and have small breasts. But the general rule is that small breasts contain a smaller amount of fat, while large breasts contain a larger amount of fat.

Fat also serves as a "shock absorber" for your delicate breast tissue as you walk, jump, run, dance, and sometimes bump into things. In general, the size of the breast gland—the part that makes and drains the milk—is similar in most breasts. That's why women with any size breasts usually can make enough breast milk to feed their babies.

Losing weight reduces the amount of fat in your body and may also make your breasts smaller. The opposite is also true: gaining weight increases your overall body fat and may make your breasts larger.

You may lose or gain weight evenly or unevenly. For example, some girls may gain weight only in their hips and thighs while their breasts stay the same. For others, their breasts may be the first place where they gain or lose weight. Others might get thin or thick all over. The position of your breasts on your chest can change as your weight goes up and down. If you lose weight in your breasts, they may sit lower on your chest or sag.

If your overall body fat is low, then you will tend to have less breast fat. If you have extra body fat, then you may have extra breast fat. Some girls have extra fat all over except in the breast area (big body but small breasts), and some girls are small all over but have big breasts (small body, big breasts). All these different combinations are normal.

Hormones and Breast Size

Your body's hormones affect your breast size too. Hormones are "bossy" chemicals made in one part of your body that go to another part of your body and tell it what to do. They turn your breast growth on, and when your breasts are finished growing they control a lot of your breast tissue's everyday activities. Estrogen and progesterone are the main hormones involved.

Just before your menstrual period starts, the hormone progesterone can make your breasts feel big and painful. When your period starts and the progesterone level falls, these symptoms ease up.

Temporary Breast Size Changes

Cold gives you goose bumps, makes your nipples and areolas get pointy, and perks your breasts up. Heat relaxes them. Lying down makes your "girls" disappear off to each side. With your arms stretched up over your head, your breasts move up with little or no sag. Bending forward at the waist can make them look narrow and long (like water bottles).

Pregnancy and breast-feeding make your breasts grow much bigger as they fill up with milk. When breast-feeding stops and all the milk is gone, they may stay bigger, return to their prior size, or become smaller. Some medications might make breasts bigger, such as some birth control pills. When you stop taking the medicine, breast size goes back to normal.

Your Age and Breast Size

Your final breast size does not depend on when they start growing. Starting to grow breasts at an early age doesn't mean you'll have big breasts, and a late start doesn't mean you'll have small ones. But once your breast growth gets going, it takes about four years to get close to their full size. Then your breasts, hips, and rear end all get rounder and wider until your early 20s. By age 25, your breasts are full-grown, even though their size and shape can still change throughout your life, for a whole lot of different reasons we've discussed, including weight gain and loss, pregnancy, breast-feeding, and medications.

girl to girl

My friend Katie started puberty before me and our other friends. In sixth grade, she was taller than me and had bigger breasts. She was very proud of them and the rest of us were pretty jealous because we were flat-chested. But now we're in eleventh grade and my breasts have grown bigger than hers. The best part about it is that now we are all happy with how our breasts turned out.

Uneven Breast Size

Lopsided breasts are pretty common, especially during puberty. Over time, they tend to even out. But like other parts of your body that come in pairs—your feet, ears, and hands—your breasts rarely become the exact same size. For no known reason, it's usually your left side that's bigger—but plenty of right breasts outsize the left.

Breast Size and Shape

Our survey of over three thousand sixth- through twelfth-grade girls and over five hundred of their moms showed that 31 percent of girls are concerned about being lopsided, but only 3 percent of moms are concerned about being uneven. This means that lopsidedness becomes less of a problem as you mature. Most of the time, your breasts tend to even out or their unevenness matters less.

There are several reasons why one breast can appear bigger than the other. The most common explanation is that there is more breast tissue on one side. Another possibility is that there is something extra *inside* the breast, like a lump or cyst (fluid-filled structure of the breast—kind of like a little water balloon). You can read more about these changes in Chapter 6. The third reason is that there is something extra *behind* the breast—like if your ribs stick out more on one side than the other. The breast sitting on the more prominent ribs can appear bigger.

Uneven-sized nipples and areolas are less common than uneven breasts. Besides size, other nipple and areola variations can occur. For example, one nipple might be pointed inward (inverted) and the other one may stick out.

Small or medium differences in breast size and shape might upset you, but probably no one else will ever notice or care. If one of your breasts is significantly bigger than the other and it really bothers you, there are things you can do to balance them out (see Chapter 8 on bras and Chapter 10 on changing breast size).

girl to girl

My right breast is slightly bigger than my left one—but the week before my period, the difference in size becomes a lot more noticeable. I get pretty self-conscious about it, but over the years I've figured out the types of bras and styles of clothing that work best to make the size difference less noticeable. It's a matter of trial and error, but it does require a bit of patience.

Narrow Breasts

Some girls have "tubular" breasts, narrow from the base out to the nipple (tube-shaped) and set far apart without any cleavage. They also tend to have a wide areola. This breast shape is not so uncommon and it carries no increased risk of any serious health problem (such as breast cancer). Most girls get comfortable with themselves and are able to find bras that give them more of a round shape.

Small Breast Size

Small breasts are very common. Think about it: you start out flat, and then all of a sudden—*boom*—breasts appear and start growing. Well, if you haven't started developing and your friends have, theirs are going to look big and yours are going to look small. Eventually yours are going to start growing too, but until they do, you might feel small. One day you might catch up and maybe even get bigger than your friends. Some girls just get growth of their nipples and areolas without any noticeable breast development underneath. It may be a timing issue: your breasts are simply not ready to grow. You might even get pubic hair and menstrual periods before any breast development. An eating disorder, such as anorexia, can be a cause of small breast size.

Large Breast Size

Girls with very big breasts can have vastly different feelings about them. Some love them and enjoy showing them off. Some love them but conceal them. Some might be okay with big breasts and have learned to live with them. But there are many who struggle with very big breasts for a number of reasons: being teased, looking top-heavy in clothes that hang over your breasts like a tent, having bra straps dig into your shoulders, getting backaches from all the extra weight in front, managing troublesome skin reactions underneath the breasts, or having difficulty playing sports because your breasts get in the way.

Size Doesn't Have to Matter

Breast growth isn't over until it's over; some girls reach their final breast size at age 16, others at age 25. Worrying does not make breasts smaller or larger, but it can consume a lot of your precious energy. No matter how big or small your breasts are, you can learn to be physically active, feel good in clothes—even a bathing suit—and be at peace in your own skin. Building your self-confidence through school-work, athletics, and outside interests, as well as developing your sense of humor, can give you the strength to deal with whatever comes your way.

Things really do get better as you get older. As your life goes on and your true personality develops, you'll see that the size of your breasts matters less and less. You will have less self-doubt and fewer hunts for body flaws. As you create your own standard for yourself, you will feel less need to compare yourself to others. Eventually, you will learn only to compare yourself to yourself—who you want to be, what you want to do, how you want to think—and that's when you'll get to enjoy the most meaningful and fun times in your life, on your own and with your friends.

girl to girl

Sounds like good advice for the future—too bad we can't be that optimistic all the time until then! Adjusting to your breast size is hard, especially when it keeps changing. Your best bet is to wear flattering clothes that fit *your* body and breasts. Try not to spend too much time dwelling on what you don't like about yourself. Say to yourself, "This is the body I have now and I'll make the best of it."

Any Questions?

We've provided answers to many of the questions that can pop up as your breast size changes.

Shouldn't my breasts be in proportion to the rest of my body?
Many of you think that everything on your body should be in proportion—all the same scale. For example, if you're tall and wide, you expect to have big and full breasts, or if you're petite, you might expect to have small breasts. But Mother Nature doesn't work that way. It's normal to have parts of your body be of different sizes. Big girls might have nice small breasts. Shorter girls might have nice large breasts.

Girls come in all different shapes and sizes with breasts that are equally unique in size and shape. Your special combination of size and form should be embraced, not "corrected."

Will my breast size be similar to the breast sizes of other women in my family?

To figure out how big your breasts will become, it's natural to check out the other women in your family. But it's not necessarily accurate. Your family's breast genes—small, medium, or large—do have a big effect on your breast size. Yet in any one family there can be a big range of sizes and shapes—small, large, and everything in between. The genetic connection also may not be obvious; breast size genes can skip around the family. You may have the same big breasts as your aunt, while your mom and sister both have small ones. So how do you know whom to compare yourself to?

The best person to look to as a predictor of your final breast size is another woman in your family who had a similar body build when she was your age (even so, your breast size still may not turn out just like hers). An older relative's *current* breast size is not a reliable predictor of your breast size. Breast size changes through life due to pregnancy, breast-feeding, menopause, and growing older. As women age they tend to gain weight all over, including in their breasts. And don't be fooled by big and loose clothes—they may hide the breasts or make them look bigger than they really are.

girl to girl

It's so interesting to look at all the different body types in my family. My aunt Eve and her 6-year-old daughter, Ella, have the same narrow, muscular body. Lena and her mom, Alice, both have long legs and feminine hips. My mom and I have different bodies—I have my dad's legs and my mom's butt—but in pictures of her when she was my age, our breasts are similar in size and shape.

Will growing taller make my breasts bigger?

Growing taller and growing breasts happen around the same time, but these two types of growth are separate. Growing taller doesn't make your breasts grow. The short growth spurt at the beginning of puberty is usually a signal that your breasts are ready to start growing. They can keep growing years after you've reached your full height. No matter how tall you become—4'11", 5'6", or 6'1"—your height has no impact on your final breast size. As we said earlier, breasts of all different sizes and shapes come on girls of all different body types.

What makes breasts sag?

A number of things can make your breasts sag. Losing weight, not wear-

ing a bra, having very large breasts, and simply getting older are some of the main reasons why breasts sag. If you don't support your breasts well enough with a bra, they will get pulled down by gravity, which causes them to sag over time. Your breasts may appear smaller when they sag because they sit lower and are more spread out over your chest. However, your breasts will generally stay the same size—they've just taken on a different shape. Anything that first makes your breasts big and then makes them small can lead to sagging—like gaining a lot of weight and then losing it, or starting and stopping breast-feeding.

How does exercise affect breast size?

Athletic girls tend to have lower overall body fat, and as a result smaller breasts. Regular physical activity keeps your body's metabolism revved up and ready for action, even when you're not exercising. The result: you burn more calories and your body fat stays lower all over, including your breasts most of the time.

Also, regular upper-body exercise makes your chest muscles bigger. When the muscles right behind your breasts (called the *pectoralis major*, or "pecs") get bigger from exercise, they push your breasts forward and can make your breasts *appear* larger. But because there are no muscles inside your breasts, exercise will not make the actual size of your breasts bigger.

How do I know if my hormones are normal or not?

Breast size is also affected by the balance of hormones that turn breast growth on and off. For example, girls who have small breasts have fewer hormones that make breasts grow and more hormones that stop breast growth. The opposite can result in big breasts: more growth-starting hormones and fewer growth-stopping ones. Size also depends on how sensitive your breast tissue is to these hormones. Breasts that are extra-sensitive to a hormone's growth signals will become bigger than breasts that pay little attention to its messages. Estrogen is the main hormone that makes breast tissue grow.

It's not possible to rush, slow down, or tip the balance of hormone signals that make your breasts grow. Your unique combination of hormones and your body's response to these hormones are already set and in general cannot be changed. If your hormones are out of balance, then you can work with your doctor to rebalance them. One example: if you have no breast growth or no periods by age sixteen, it may be because your hormones are slow to get going. Your doctor can check out your hormone levels, then either leave things alone or suggest a little "nudge" to speed things up. Another example: you may notice a lot of extra body hair and irregular periods. This might go along with lower levels of female hormones and higher levels of male hormones than the average girl. Your doctor can help you manage this.

Big differences in hormone activity from one person to another are normal. You can't see your hormones, but you and your doctor can see how your hormones are working based on all of the changes of puberty that are visible and measurable—like your menstrual cycle. If you think you have a problem with your hormones, talk to your parents and your doctor. Your doctor can check your hormone levels to make sure that everything is okay.

Are there hormones in food that affect breast size?

Breasts are getting bigger than ever before for a bunch of reasons: more people are overweight, breast-enlarging surgery is more common, and hormones in our food may make breasts grow larger.

Some foods and drinks may contain substances that might act like your own body's natural hormones but cause extra unhealthy breast growth. These substances include:

- Hormones, given to animals to make them grow bigger faster or produce more milk

- Hormone-like chemicals found in some commonly used plastic containers

- Certain fertilizers, which make plants grow faster

- Some pesticides that protect fruits, vegetables, and grains from insects

Small amounts of these ingredients can remain on or in the food you eat. A little bit here or there is probably harmless, but people who eat a lot of foods that contain these chemicals

girl to girl

Hormones in food...sounds scary, huh? When I first heard about these things, I got worried about what's in my food too. The best thing we can do is to limit the amount of fast food and junk we eat. Craving something crunchy? Try a carrot, a rice cake, or nuts instead of chips. How about something sweet? Have a bunch of organic grapes or an apple. To make sure you have the right food at home, ask your mom or dad to buy more organic food the next time she or he goes grocery shopping. Taking control of your diet is more empowering than you may think.

over many years may experience extra growth in their bodies and maybe in their breasts. Thinking of eating more foods with hormones to make your breasts bigger? Bad idea! Making an effort to consume more of these hormones or substances is very unhealthy and will cause more harm than good. A better idea is to change to a healthier diet. Right away, anyone can improve her health by choosing and preparing foods carefully. In Chapter 12, we'll give you plenty of tips to help you do this.

Will I stay flat forever?
There is nothing wrong with you if you have very small breasts or your chest appears relatively flat. Try to be patient with your body's pace of growth. Later in life, your breasts might still get bigger. Pregnancy makes flat or very small breasts bigger. Your breasts are a part of you; they don't define you or make you a better or worse person.

If you want your breasts to appear bigger, there are a lot of things that you can do. We have a whole section in this book (in Chapter 9) on how to present yourself in ways that make you feel better.

girl to girl

Sometimes I wish I had small breasts like my good friend Sam. She's petite and can wear whatever she wants and it almost never looks too revealing. There are some clothes that look awesome on her that I could never pull off.

If someone has suffered from anorexia, will that affect their breast size?
Girls with the eating disorder anorexia usually have very small breasts. The production of the hormones that turn on breast development and bring on menstrual periods slows or stops in girls who are super-thin. The growth of the milk-making tissue in the breasts shuts down or doesn't get a chance to start. Fat is lost in all parts of the body, including the breasts.

Breasts will stay very small in girls who remain very thin. Weight gain increases the amount of fat in the breasts, making them bigger. Also, weight gain increases the hormones responsible for breast development, enlarging the breasts.

Breast Size and Shape

Breast size may return to normal if the breast gland inside had a chance to develop. But if a girl stays very thin during much of puberty, the chance to develop breasts might be partially missed, and breast size might not be able to catch up all the way.

Many girls want to be thin so they can feel stylish. But sometimes girls lose too much weight and don't know when to stop. This is a serious problem that requires immediate help. If you are in this situation, talk to your parents or someone you trust and get help right away. The sooner you overcome this problem and recover, the healthier you'll be. This is a "now" problem, not a "later" one.

How do I deal with really big breasts?

Over time, you will come up with all kinds of solutions, tricks, and tips for dealing with the extra needs that go along with very big breasts. And we're here to help you. Our book has special sections on presenting yourself to the world, including wearing the best clothes to flatter your body, finding the best bras for support and comfort, reducing back pain and improving your posture, and preventing and treating skin rashes.

You can share your stories at TakingCareOfYourGirls.com.

I thought I felt a lump once, but it was just because I had my period. My mother, who's a school nurse, checked to make sure.

Trisha, 17

What's That?

3

Noticing, Feeling, and Checking for Breast Changes

When should you start getting regular breast examinations?

Amanda, 15

I don't ask a lot of questions for a few reasons: (1) I'm afraid everyone already knows the answer and I'm just naive. (2) If no one else is asking questions, I feel awkward being the only one asking. (3) It's sort of a private topic that I'm not used to talking about out loud.

Delia, 16

I went up two sizes over summer break! I started seventh grade with a C cup. Then my breasts got these weird pink stripes on the side. What happened?

Veronica, 12

My aunt Toni just got diagnosed with breast cancer. Does that mean I'm going to get it too? Should I be feeling for changes?

Claire, 16

The most disgusting thing happened to me ever. I got a huge zit on my breast—just in time for tank-top season! I thought breasts would be a trouble-free skin zone—no freckles, no zits.

Alix, 20

I am in fifth grade and my mom wants to have a talk with me about breast self-examination. But I don't want to talk about it. I'm still wearing a training bra and I don't think I need to know that stuff yet.

Sydney, 10

I got a rash all over my breasts right before prom night. I tried to put base makeup on it and that just made it worse.

Ashanti, 18

I have no idea how I'm supposed to know what a lump would feel like or even where I should look for one.

Rowanda, 15

All of a sudden my breasts feel so sore. I know if I tell my mom, she'll freak. And I really can't deal with some strange doctor giving me an exam.

Samara, 13

I heard my mom joke with her friend that when she gets a mammogram they won't be able to even see everything because her breasts are huge. But I don't think it's funny. What if she's right? What if they can't see everything?

Maddy, 11

My friend and I thought it would be fun to sunbathe nude on her building's rooftop. I got a sunburn right on my breasts. It itched so bad I couldn't wear a bra.

Aaliyah, 20

What's That?

My breasts feel kind of irregular, so I can never tell what feels like an actual lump or what's just another part of my breast. I wish I had more information!

Toni, 16

As my breasts grow I know I need to examine them to make sure there is nothing wrong. But my mom says I am too young to be worried about breast cancer.

Keisha, 14

I heard that women have to have a mammogram every year of their lives after 40. But I wonder if that is true if you have really small breasts.

Britney, 15

First Things First

As your breasts grow and mature, you'll notice all kinds of changes along the way. You can expect changes on the outside and on the inside; you or your doctor may discover these changes as your breasts develop. Maybe you felt something by accident—say, someone bumped into you and that area felt painful, and then you touch it and just happen to find some lumps and bumps. Or maybe you feel something unusual while soaping yourself in the shower.

This chapter is the place to find out how you can look, see, feel, and find changes in your breasts. Then the next four chapters will explain different kinds of changes you might discover on the inside and the outside of the breast. You'll be amazed by how much more you'll know after you have finished these chapters, especially about what's within the realm of normal. The more you know about your body, the better you'll feel about dealing with its changes.

Here's the Scoop

Noticing New Things

When you get dressed in the morning, undress at night, and hop in and out of the shower or tub, you might notice outside changes on your breasts: stretch marks, bug bites, sunburn, rashes, breakouts, bumps and bruises, freckles, or other spots. Nipple and areola changes might also happen as your breasts develop: darkening color, sprouting nipple hairs, and leaking a little bit of fluid from the nipple. Sometimes it's hard to remember if what you're seeing or feeling has been there all along or if it's something new.

Other changes can be more dramatic. For example, you might notice that your breasts are getting bigger very quickly.

Feeling New Feelings

Growing breasts commonly produce strange new feelings: tingling, shooting pains, aches, burning, itching, throbbing, crawling sensation, fullness, heaviness, tightness. Some of these changes are like "growing pains" and some are due to the ups and downs of your hormones during your menstrual cycle. New sensations can also result from ordinary day-to-day things that happen to you—like getting bumped, doing strenuous upper-body exercise, consuming certain foods and drinks, or taking some medicines.

Looking for Changes: Breast Self-Exam or Your Doctor's Examination

If you don't love the idea of examining your own breasts, you're not alone. A lot of girls—women, too—worry that they don't know when to do it, how to do it, and what to look and feel for. Many girls say that *everything* feels like a lump and it's hard to know what's normal or what's not. But learning the right technique and getting in the habit of performing regular breast checks can help. With practice, you'll become familiar with the "neighborhoods" of your breasts and what's normal *for you*. Then it's easier to recognize a change or something new that stands out that you don't remember feeling before.

There is more than one "right" way to *examine your own breasts*. The most important thing is to look over and feel through all of both breasts: from top to bottom, side to side, and front to back.

girl to girl

I thought you only did breast exams to look for breast cancer. I was totally wrong! Doing a breast self-exam is just a way of getting to know this part of your body. The better you know your body, the better you'll be able to notice any kind of change . . . which is most often *not* breast cancer.

The first part of the exam is where you do a careful inspection. Stand in front of a mirror and look carefully over both breasts in two positions: with your hands on your hips, then with your hands above your head. Notice the shapes of your two breasts in both positions. Check the skin for color changes, rashes, pimples, and spots, and look for any changes in shape and size, dimples, dents, bulges, and unevenness.

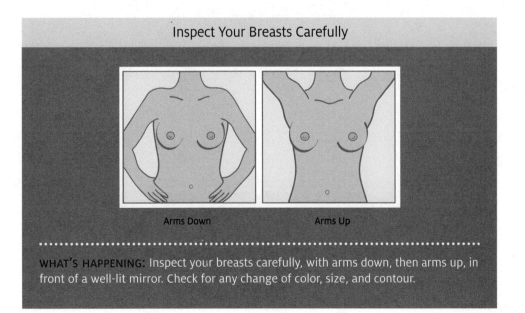

Inspect Your Breasts Carefully

Arms Down   Arms Up

WHAT'S HAPPENING: Inspect your breasts carefully, with arms down, then arms up, in front of a well-lit mirror. Check for any change of color, size, and contour.

Breast self-exams are like getting to know two close friends very, very well ☺. Examine each breast with your opposite hand: your right hand examines your left breast, the left hand checks out your right breast. With the flat pads (where your fingerprints are) of your three middle fingers together, use a circular motion to examine all of both breasts.

The next step is to feel throughout each breast in two positions: sitting or standing up and lying down. You can do this part of the self-exam in your bed, bathtub, or shower. It all comes down to *examining yourself wherever you feel most comfortable.* The shower or bath has a built-in advantage because the water and soap make your fingers slide over your breasts more easily. Plus it's a quick add-on to the washing you're already doing.

Feel the front to the back of each breast by slightly increasing the amount of pressure you apply. Use a light touch to feel the breast tissue closest to the surface of your skin, a firm touch for the middle section of breast tissue, and a bit more pressure to feel the deepest breast tissue.

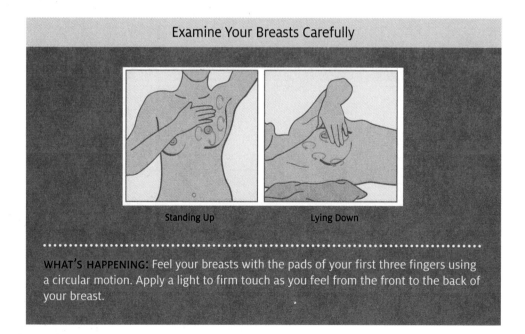

Examine Your Breasts Carefully

Standing Up

Lying Down

WHAT'S HAPPENING: Feel your breasts with the pads of your first three fingers using a circular motion. Apply a light to firm touch as you feel from the front to the back of your breast.

Two Ways to Examine All of Both Breasts

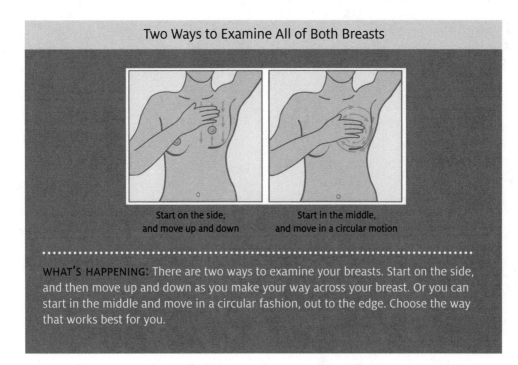

Start on the side,
and move up and down

Start in the middle,
and move in a circular motion

WHAT'S HAPPENING: There are two ways to examine your breasts. Start on the side, and then move up and down as you make your way across your breast. Or you can start in the middle and move in a circular fashion, out to the edge. Choose the way that works best for you.

There are two patterns of examination you could use. It's important to use one pattern to examine both breasts completely during each examination.

- Move your fingers horizontally up and down your breast, like you're mowing a lawn.

- Move your fingers around in a spiral direction, starting from the nipple and circling out towards the edge of your breast.

As long as you cover your breasts entirely, both methods work equally well. It's important to pay attention during your exam. Try not to be distracted by other things that may be on your mind.

Look and feel for anything that stands out from or feels different than the majority of your breast tissue. Remember the *Sesame Street* lesson "One of these things is not like the other"? When you're examining

The first time I felt a lump, I got really worried. I went to the doctor and it turned out to be nothing—just a variation in my normal breast terrain. I know, my mom's a doctor—so why did I go see someone else? Because when I have a breast issue, I'd rather have my mom's support and reassurance than her medical advice. If *you* feel a specific lump in your breast, don't worry. Nearly always, lumps in girls' breasts are nothing serious. Did you know that over 99 percent of breast lumps in girls under age 20 are benign—meaning not cancerous? But rather than think about it too much, have your doctor check it out.

your breasts, one area might feel like a mountain range, another area might feel like a rocky road, another region like a sandy beach, a bunch of grapes, or a bag of marbles. In each neighborhood, see if you can feel something that's different from the rest of the breast tissue. For example, if you feel a big rock on the sandy beach or a peanut in a bowl of oatmeal and it does not go away, let your doctor know. It's probably perfectly normal, but it's still best to check it out.

Your Doctor's Exam

Getting a breast exam by your doctor can feel strange and embarrassing. There's no doubt about it—the whole idea of being examined by a stranger takes courage and a lot of getting used to. But it's just one of those things that we girls and women have to do to stay healthy.

Breast examination is usually taken one step at a time. First, start getting familiar with your breasts by examining them regularly. Some girls examine their breasts once a month, but most girls do it every few months—both are fine. Your pediatrician or nurse practitioner will check your breasts during your yearly visit. Later, when you get a bit older, your routine breast examinations will be done by a gynecologist (a doctor who specializes in women's health).

If you feel or see something that concerns you in between your routine doctor visits, make a special appointment to get it checked out. Your regular doctor can usually handle most issues. You might prefer a dermatologist (skin doctor) to deal with breakouts, rashes, spots, or unwanted hair. Your regular doctor may send you to a breast specialist if she or he thinks the breast concern at hand should be looked at further.

To keep a closer watch on any area of concern, your doctor will probably schedule another breast exam in a few weeks or months, depending on your situation. Sometimes a breast test may be recommended on one or both sides to check out a breast change that you or your doctor might have seen or felt.

girl to girl

The first time I went for a checkup after my breasts started growing, I was so nervous. To make matters even worse, my doctor was a man! Wow—how embarrassing. I just kept saying over and over in my head, *He does this every day. He does this every day. He does this every day. . . .*

Tests on Breasts

Some of the following tests may be familiar to you. Most of the time they are used for older women. But sometimes these tests can be very helpful in checking out a breast finding in girls.

- ULTRASOUND is the most common test used to evaluate something you might feel in your breast. This test helps see if a lump is a ball of breast tissue or a sac of fluid. It also gathers important information about the size, shape, and contour of the lump.

  An ultrasound is a very simple test that's done in a doctor's office or a radiology department. A small amount of gel is put on the breast and then a handheld device that emits sound waves (it sort of looks like a TV remote) is moved over the skin surface. A computer tracks how the sound waves pass through the breast tissue and creates a picture of the inside of the breast.

  This test doesn't hurt, but occasionally it might be a little uncomfortable if the handheld device is cold or pushes up against a tender spot.

- MAMMOGRAMS are pictures of the breasts used to detect breast cancer. They are rarely done in women under age 20 because in such young women, breast cancer is so, so rare and it's very hard to see through the dense breast gland tissue normally present in young women. When you get to age 40, you'll need to get a mammogram each year. If women in your family have been diagnosed with breast cancer under age 50, then you would start getting mammograms earlier than age 40. The general rule is you start getting mammograms 10 years younger than the age of the youngest person in your family affected by breast cancer. For example, if your mom had breast cancer at age 42, then you'd start getting yearly mammograms at age 32.

- MAGNETIC RESONANCE IMAGING (MRI) is a fancy test that can be used to take pictures of the breasts. MRI is not a routine test. It's only used to carefully evaluate an area of concern that has already been checked out by an ultrasound (or sometimes even a mammogram).

   An MRI is very helpful as a watching tool for women over 18 with a strong family history of breast cancer (strong means that several women in the family have had breast cancer, particularly at a relatively young age; men in your family have had breast cancer; or there's a breast cancer gene in the family). MRI is also used for women diagnosed with breast cancer.

- NIPPLE FLUID TEST Some girls might get a little fluid coming out of their nipples, on one or both sides. This fluid should be tested for blood and for cells, normal or otherwise. Your doctor can collect the fluid, put it on a slide, and examine it under a microscope. Sometimes your breast might need to be massaged or squeezed a little bit to get enough fluid to come out for inspection.

- FLUID REMOVAL from the breasts can also be called *needle aspiration.* (This has nothing to do with fluid you might have noticed coming out of the nipple.) If you have a lump in your breast that looks like a simple cyst (a fluid-filled, round structure) based on an ultrasound test, nothing more is usually done. But if the cyst is causing a problem (like pain or pressure) and if the problem is not going away on its own, then your doctor might recommend removing the fluid in the cyst to relieve your symptoms. The fluid is removed with a thin needle and then checked out under the microscope.

An *aspiration* or *biopsy* might be recommended every once in a while to see if an area of concern is made up of normal or abnormal cells. A fine-needle aspiration obtains a few cells for inspection under a microscope, using a thin needle and a syringe. A thicker needle can remove a small core of tissue for evaluation. To take out a bigger piece of tissue, a surgeon can make a small incision in the skin through which he or she will remove the tissue. Numbing medicine is used to avoid pain during a biopsy. You will be left with a small scar after a biopsy, but the incision will lighten, flatten, and become barely visible over time.

You can share the information here to help the women in your family get the medical tests they need. If they need more information on tests, check out www.breastcancer.org.

Any Questions?

What's the best time of the month to examine yourself?
Examine your breasts a week or two after your period starts. Around your period, your breasts can become big, tender, and extra lumpy. Don't examine your breasts at that time—it will drive you crazy!

girl to girl

I've observed some of these procedures at my mom's hospital and they are really no big deal. The doctors who perform them know exactly what they are doing and try to make the process as comfortable as possible. I'd say that the worst part about the whole procedure is the anxiety you feel leading up to it. The anticipation usually feels worse than the actual thing you're dreading.

How often should I do breast self-exams?
Get in the habit of examining your breasts every month. Try to do the exams around the same time each month. If your period is irregular and skips a few months, pick a day in each month to perform your exams. For instance, you could do a self-exam on the first of each month.

I have breast cancer in my family. Do I have to examine myself more often?
For girls, the risk of breast cancer is nearly zero, even if you have a number of family members who've had it. The main purpose of you and your doctor examining your breasts starting early on is to become familiar with your breasts' unique "terrain" and to get in the healthy habit of checking your breasts over the course of your life. Your doctor will do an exam once a year, which is just as often as anyone else gets it done. No routine tests are done in your teens.

Past your teens, into your 20s, your doctor might add a breast test (like a mammogram and MRI) to your regular follow-up plan, depending on your situation and your family history.

Of course, along the way, if you note any lasting change in the way your breasts look or feel, be sure to show your doctor.

How is my breast exam going to change as my breasts get bigger?
The bigger your breasts grow, the more breast tissue you'll have to feel during your exams. On the outside, you might notice skin changes such as stretch marks, darkening of the areola and/or nipple, and sometimes nipple hair. On the inside, new growth can add to the regular mix of lumps and bumps that you might feel.

How do you remember what your breasts feel like from month to month?
Have trouble remembering what your breasts feel like and what things are new or the same? That's true for most of us. Simple solution: keep a journal to record your findings from month to month. Any notebook

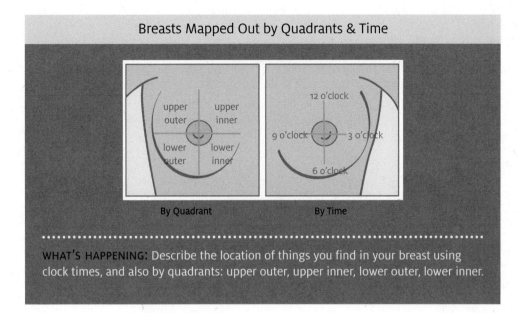

Breasts Mapped Out by Quadrants & Time

upper outer | upper inner
lower outer | lower inner

By Quadrant

12 o'clock
9 o'clock — 3 o'clock
6 o'clock

By Time

WHAT'S HAPPENING: Describe the location of things you find in your breast using clock times, and also by quadrants: upper outer, upper inner, lower outer, lower inner.

will do. Be sure to date the journal entry and indicate in which part of your breast you find anything. It might be helpful to draw a diagram.

Once you've drawn a picture of each breast, you can describe the location of the thing you see or feel using the clock. For example, the upper outer area of the right breast goes from 12:00 to 3:00. The lower outer area of the right breast goes from 3:00 to 6:00, the lower inner area goes from 6:00 to 9:00, and the upper inner area is from 9:00 to 12:00. The opposite is true for the left side. For example, you might note in the left upper outer quadrant, in the 2:00 position, a cluster of grape-like lumps that are about half an inch (1 centimeter) each and that wiggle around a little.

What kind of doctor does a biopsy?

Any breast surgery should be done by a doctor who specializes in breast procedures. For a fine-needle aspiration or a needle or core biopsy, a breast radiologist or a breast surgeon is the best type of doctor to go to. Both are experts in the diagnosis of breast problems.

If you ever were to need a biopsy that involves a small incision (cut in the skin), the size and placement of the incision is very important. An experienced breast surgeon knows how to stay away from the nerves of the breast so your breast sensation remains normal, and how to hide an incision so it doesn't show when you wear a bathing suit or tank top. Incisions along the tops of the breasts, particularly in the middle, tend to show and not disappear very well, so you want to avoid that location if possible.

How do I know if a lump needs to be removed or should be left alone?
If there is a lump in the center of your breast—one side or both—and if your breasts are still growing, that lump is probably part of your breast bud responsible for giving rise to your breast tissue. The lump should not be removed because it might interfere with your normal breast development. If you are concerned about any recommended treatment (or lack thereof) prescribed by your doctor, be sure to see a breast care specialist for an experienced judgment before following through with a procedure.

I'm nervous about getting the breast test that my doctor recommended.
It's completely normal to be worried about any medical test. No one likes the inconvenience, waiting, uncertainty, discomfort, and anxiety. Try to ignore all these annoying things. Bring something to read and music to listen to while you wait. Know that the test will be over very quickly. When the test is over, pat yourself on the back for going out of your way to take good care of yourself!

You can share your stories at TakingCareOfYourGirls.com.

Skin Stuff:

4

Stretch Marks, Breakouts, Rashes

There are little whiteheads on my areolas. I don't know what they are. Is it bad to pop them?

Hailey, 14

My favorite thing to do is lie on the beach in the sun with my friends during the summer (with bathing suits, of course). I don't burn, I tan. That's not going to make me more likely to get breast cancer, is it?

Brittany, 16

My breasts *finally* started to grow, after waiting a *very* long time. They were looking very nice until I got these pink puffy stretch marks on the sides. I am so upset. I never want anyone to see them, ever, not even my friends—they are so ugly.

Dana, 13

I found some special cream in my mom's bathroom for stretch marks. Can I use it on my breasts? The bottle doesn't say anything about being okay for breasts and I'm not about to ask anyone about it.

Anna, 15

I have red hair and pale, freckly skin, so I've always used a ton of sunscreen. But I forgot to put it on once and got a sunburn above and between my breasts. *Sooo* painful!

Sage, 12

When I play soccer, I have to wear two sports bras to keep my breasts from jiggling. But they squoosh my breasts together, and then afterward, when I take the bras off, I often break out in between my breasts. It's terrible! What am I doing wrong?

Hope, 16

In the summer, I get really annoying red rashes under both my breasts, making it very hard to wear a bra. It never goes away completely until the middle of winter, and I'm too embarrassed to show anyone. It's so frustrating!

Tanya, 14

The weirdest thing happened. I got the nicest tan during my vacation, and then, just about a week later, pale round spots showed up at the bottom of my neck down to the upper part of my breasts. They went from pink to white. *What are they?*

Melanie, 19

There's a birthmark on the side of my left breast that's getting bigger and darker as my breast grows. I'm scared.

Theresa, 12

First Things First

As your breasts grow, you may notice little and big skin changes on them: stretch marks, rashes, acne, hair, freckles, birthmarks, sunburns, and more. You might wonder what changes are okay and which you need to be concerned about, how long they will last, and what will make them go away. Keep reading for some helpful answers *and* some ways you can start protecting your "girls" today.

Here's the Scoop

Stretch Marks

Most teenagers get stretch marks on their breasts, belly and hip areas—the round areas of the body. When you're growing really quickly, such as during puberty, stretch marks can appear. Your skin can't expand fast enough to cover the expansion underneath, and it gets over-stressed. Little tears occur in the bottom layer of your skin, called the *dermis,* resulting in stretch marks.

Some girls are more prone to stretch marks than others. Genes that run in your family can affect how stiff or elastic your skin is, how fast your body and its curves grow, and thus your tendency to get stretch marks.

When stretch marks first show up, you might not know what they are. They first appear as pink, red, purple, or silvery lines, sometimes slightly raised above the skin. They can appear solo or in groups lined up next to each other like a stack of pancakes with a little space in between each one. Over time—say, six months to a few years—the marks get smaller, flatter, and paler. Eventually, they may appear lighter than your own skin color. By the time you're an adult, you can hardly see them unless you look extra-hard or get up real close.

Sunburn

The chest area tends to get a *lot* of sun exposure over the years—in tank tops, bathing suits, sundresses, and so on. While the sun feels really good, it's quite harmful to your skin. It's very important to protect yourself—especially the chest area—from the sun using sunscreen and proper clothing. While sunbathing, your skin is being exposed to harmful ultraviolet (UV) rays that damage the skin. Look around at older women who have tons of freckles and "age spots"; that's from years and years of heavy sun exposure before effective sunscreen was so easily available. Too much sun exposure can also lead to skin cancer. Tanning salons are especially unhealthy because they expose you to highly concentrated UV rays. If you like a bronzed look, self-tanning solutions are much safer. See this chapter's "Any Questions?" section for more about sun protection.

girl to girl

In my freshman year of high school, I ran indoor track during the winter and wore a sports bra that was *way* too small for me. The bra gave decent support only because it smooshed my boobs together so tightly they couldn't move! Anyway, between the chest sweat and boob friction from all the exercise, I developed a little rash on my chest. I started applying a pure steroid cream (used to get rid of rashes and inflammation) to the rash . . . bad idea! Within a week, the whole area on which I had applied the cream had completely erupted with a horrible, red, bumpy breakout. I went to the dermatologist, who told me that the steroid cream had aggravated the little patch of acne I thought was a rash. She gave me the correct acne treatment, and within a few weeks my "rackne"—a name a friend gave to this type of acne—cleared up.

Acne or Breakouts

Acne is common between and under your breasts. Wearing an athletic bra during sports can bring about breakouts pretty often. The combination of skin against skin, sweat, heat, rubbing, and a lack of airflow is a setup for breakouts. Since supporting your breasts is so important, especially when you're active, don't let breakouts be a reason for you not to wear a sports bra. There is a lot you can do to avoid and get rid of breakouts.

Skin Stuff

To keep your breasts clean and acne-free, it's important to shower immediately after sports, dry your skin off carefully, wash and dry your bra after each use, and try to avoid having skin rub against skin, like under and between your breasts. Dust baby powder made of cornstarch (not talc, because it's unsafe to breathe in the talc dust that gets into the air) around your breasts and under your arms to help absorb some of the moisture, reduce friction, and soothe your skin. If you already have breakouts: no squeezing or scrubbing, and no steroid creams. Go visit your doctor for special wash solutions, and possibly antibiotics. A lot of times, the same acne creams and washes used for faces can be used to treat chest acne.

Rashes

Rashes can happen to anyone at any age, not just to babies. A rash is a change of the skin's color, look, and feel due to some sort of irritation. The color can be pale pink, red, or brown; the texture can be flat, bumpy, or both; and the rash can have smooth, round, or irregular edges.

A rash can be caused by an allergic reaction to a new medication (such as an antibiotic), a new product (a new detergent used to wash your clothes or a new lotion you're using), or something from nature (poison ivy or nettles). You can get a rash from an infection, from the sun, or from skin rubbing together.

In the cleavage area or under your breasts, rashes, acne, infection, and other forms of skin irritation are all more likely to happen. That's because the extra warmth, moisture, darkness, and friction inside skin folds and creases is a setup for infection and irritation. Bottom line: skin does not like to be up against skin.

Any rash can itch and cause a smell that usually only you are aware of. You don't want to scratch because that could leave a scar. The best way to get rid of the itch or smell is to treat the cause of the rash. Solutions depend on what type of rash you have.

Chafing

You can get tiny scratches, pinkness, and irritation when a wet bathing suit or bra chafes your skin. A bra that fits shouldn't rub. When you play sports, use an athletic bra that supports your breasts without rubbing. If you have a bra that rubs in a specific spot, find the problem area and try to fix it. If the tag is rubbing, cut it off. If there is a rough seam or stiff thread, see what you can do to soften it up. You can also sew a piece of an old, soft cotton T-shirt over that area. During athletics, some girls wear a soft cotton tank top *under* their bra, then another T-shirt on top over their bra. To protect the nipples from rubbing, some girls use an extra-large Band-Aid (get one that's ouchless to remove).

Birthmarks and Freckles

As you grow, your spots can grow too. Spots you've always had on your breasts may change and make you concerned. Birthmarks can get bigger and bumpier, change colors, and sprout hair.

Few of these changes ever become a problem. Small changes in the shape and size of birthmarks are common—but it's still important to show your doctor during your regular visits. Big size and color changes should be checked out right away to make sure everything is okay and so a doctor can answer any questions you might have. Any hair that's growing can be cut carefully with the tip of a very small pair of scissors.

Freckles, those ordinary little flat brown spots on your skin, might be all over your body or just in a few places. It's pretty common to get them on the upper part of your breasts in the middle of your chest, from sun exposure. Over time, you may notice more of them. Freckles are nothing to worry about unless you see a significant change. If a freckle takes on new colors; gets wider, thicker, or more irregular; or forms a raw area on top, have your doctor check things out.

Yeast Infections

You've probably heard of or experienced yeast infections of the vagina or vulva (very common and very treatable). But did you know that when you head up north to the "breast department," yeast infections are quite common on your skin in that area?

Yeast is a tiny one-celled organism that belongs to the fungus family. A small amount of yeast exists on every human being. But when the balance of yeast and bacteria on the skin is thrown off, it can result in a yeast infection, often showing up as a rash.

Yeast's favorite place to hang out is in the warm, dark, and moist environment inside skin folds. Yeast infections are different from acne (or "rackne"). They can show up as irregular patches of pink and red bumps scattered around a certain area or grouped together in one cluster. The rash can itch, burn, and cause a mild odor that usually only you can smell. Girls with large breasts are more prone to this kind of yeast infection because the breasts naturally rest against the top of the belly wall. The pressure and rubbing of a big bra band under both breasts can make matters worse. You can also get a breakout of acne between your breasts in the middle of a yeast infection (see treatment suggestions in the Q&A).

There's another type of skin yeast infection that can appear on your upper chest area, back, and arms in clusters of round spots that are about $\frac{1}{4}$ inch in diameter and are slightly rough on the surface. They usually start out light pink and then become paler than the surrounding skin, but sometimes they turn light brown. The pale spots are more noticeable on girls with dark or tan skin. A fancy name for this type of yeast infection is *tinea versicolor.* Unlike with other types of yeast infections, you should go directly to a dermatologist if you suspect you have tinea versicolor. Your doctor may recommend treatment with a lotion (over-the-counter miconazole) or a special shampoo (Selsun Blue or Nizoral) regularly for a week or so. To keep the rash from coming back, ongoing treatment is necessary. Occasionally a pill might be prescribed for a few days. It may take a few weeks or months for the skin color to even out completely and return to normal.

Not to worry—yeast infections are not contagious. That means that you can't catch them from somebody or spread them to someone else. But if you think you have a yeast infection, see your doctor or nurse practitioner for help. Some common treatments are described in the "Any Questions?" section.

Bumps and Bruises

Sometimes your breasts get bumped and bruised as you run around, play sports, or battle your brothers or sisters. Most knocks don't leave any mark, but a big bump can injure tiny blood vessels, causing a little blood to leak under the skin. The resulting bruise can make your skin go from black and blue to yellow, green, then pink. Nothing bad will arise from a bruise on your breast. When everything heals, your skin will return to its normal color.

Any Questions?

How can I prevent or get rid of stretch marks?
You can't keep stretch marks from happening or take them away once they're there. But the good news is that stretch marks get better on their own over time. Until then, you can use tinted lotions to even out your skin color if they bother you.

Save your money and don't buy those expensive creams that promise to remove stretch marks. They don't really work since they are absorbed only into the surface of your skin, not down into the bottom layer where stretch marks occur. Retin-A, acid washes, and laser therapy are not recommended because they are unlikely to work, have unpleasant side effects, and are expensive.

What kind of sunscreen should I use?
Nowadays, there are various strengths of sunscreen available that block both types of harmful sun rays, UVA and UVB, and can last for many hours in the sun. The higher the sun protection factor (SPF) number of the sunscreen, the stronger the sunblock. Don't be afraid to get the highest SPF product you can. They now come as high as 50 or 70 SPF, and each year they get higher as the products improve. Even though a summer tan looks great temporarily, you have to take care of your skin in the long term. Most dermatologists recommend a sunscreen of at least SPF 30 that will block most of the sun's harmful rays, but you can still get some color. Don't use anything less than this because it won't block enough of the harmful UV rays. No matter what lotion you use, you still have to be careful about how much time you spend in the sun.

Be careful to apply the sunscreen to all skin areas at least twenty minutes before you go out in the sun. Most lotions need this time to be absorbed into your skin, so they can be most effective. If you skip some areas, it could lead to interesting and undesirable splotches of burned skin.

How can I make the breakouts between my breasts go away?
You can definitely deal with acne or breakouts around your breasts, but you should know that breakouts on the breasts are treated a bit differently than those on the face. For example, some of the medications that are used on the face (such as Retin-A) can be too drying for the breasts. Washes containing benzoyl peroxide can be effective and are available over the counter at many pharmacies. These can help to remove excess oils, act as an antibiotic to kill germs on the skin, and prevent the pores from clogging up. If you can't get to a shower right away after exercising, cleanse your chest area using wipes containing

benzoyl peroxide. These wipes are available without a prescription at your local pharmacy and can easily fit in your gym bag. Be aware that any of these products that are left on the skin can bleach your clothing, so wearing a white T-shirt may be your best bet.

If your problem does not improve after two weeks of using these products, make an appointment to see a dermatologist. He or she can help you with stronger prescription medications.

A dermatologist will usually prescribe a wash and an antibiotic cream that's applied to the skin. Some girls may require oral medications (taken by mouth), especially if there are breakouts in other areas such as the face or back.

You may be tempted to try to scrub away the breakouts. Don't do it! Picking at and scrubbing acne just leads to soreness, can make the breakout take longer to heal, and may even leave permanent scars. Mild cleansers with soft beads may be okay, but only if you are very gentle in how you use them.

How do I get rid of yeast infections around my breasts?

The first step in treating a yeast infection is addressing what caused it. That means keeping the affected area clean and dry and making sure there are stretches of time without skin-to-skin contact when you can air out the area. As soon as you get out of the bath or shower, dry your skin well. Next, dust that area with baby powder (again, make sure it's made of cornstarch, not talc).

girl to girl

If having a yeast infection gives me an excuse to take off my bra and walk around topless in my bedroom (with the door locked—I have two brothers), it sounds like a pretty good exchange to me.

When you're out and about, wear a bra that lifts and separates your breasts, and that dries quickly if you tend to sweat. At home, take your bra off and put a folded or rolled-up towel under your breasts to prevent skin-to-skin contact and get some air circulation. Or just pick your "girls" up under a loose shirt and let the air flow around them. You can even set a hair dryer on cool (not warm or hot) and blow air over the area.

If you get a little pink under your breasts regularly, dust the area with an over-the-counter antifungal powder. If you have a real rash that's definitely from a yeast infection, you'll need to use an antifungal cream.

There are many options available over the counter in your drugstore, such as lotrimin. *Do not use a steroid-only cream, such as Cortaid or other brand of cortisone, because steroids alone can make a yeast infection worse, not better.*

If the rash is really bothering you or it hasn't gotten better with over-the-counter preparations after one to two weeks, go see a dermatologist to make sure that it is truly a yeast infection. The rash could be due to something else.

If your doctor says it's a yeast infection, he or she will probably prescribe a stronger cream or ointment that combines an anti-yeast medicine with a steroid to help make the redness, swelling, and itching go away.

You can share your stories at TakingCareOfYourGirls.com.

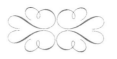

Once I was using a tissue to smooth the protrusion of my nipple from my shirt and I didn't realize that you could see the tissue. Of course, it looked like I was trying to make my boobs look bigger. My mom asked me about it, and already embarrassed, I couldn't face saying the word "nipple" in front of her, so I agreed that I was trying to use the tissue as a boob boost.

Melanie, 15

Nipple Tips: 5

Itches, Fluid, Hair, Inverted, and Other Stuff

Here's something you never hear people talking about. I had extra breast tissue under my armpit area that I first noticed in fifth grade. It seemed like a lump, and when I showed my mom, she made an appointment with our doctor right away. I didn't know it at the time, but we have a family history of breast cancer, so Mom must have been freaking. But she acted calm, so I never really worried. It turned out to be nothing, just extra tissue. It's just one of those things, but of course when you're 10, you want to be exactly like every other girl.

Sari, 18

Why do some girls get hair around their breasts? Actually, why do *I* have hair there? I knew I would get pubic hair, but not this! Is it normal or something I should be worried about?

Jess, 13

Do nipples get much bigger when breasts are fully developed?

Keiko, 10

I told a "friend" that I had a nipple hair. Next thing I know, I'm walking down the hall at school and the captain of the football team says, "Hey, nipple hair, how's it going?" I could have *just died*!

Molly, 17

I have larger nipples than most girls. When I'm wearing a thin-cup bra, it looks like I have lumps on top of my breasts!

Vanessa, 16

My sister's and my mom's nipples stick out like they're supposed to. But mine stick in. I thought that was supposed to be genetic.

Robin, 19

I asked my mom why her nipples pointed down. That did not make her happy!

Patricia, 12

One of my friends felt bad about the black hair around her areola, thinking she couldn't do anything about it. She grew up with her dad and didn't feel comfortable asking him, so I became her confidante.

Jenny, 19

Right in the middle of French, this boy started laughing and pointing at my breasts. I looked down and saw why—it was like you could see right through my shirt to my nipples. I wanted to die of embarrassment!

Alix, 13

My nipples sometimes leak! Is that breast milk?

Brianna, 11

My best friend told me that she had "nipple envy." She wished she could have tiny nipples like mine, but her areolas are really dark and big. I told her I wish I had bigger breasts like hers. I wonder if we're weird to talk about this stuff!

Nikki, 14

My brother threw a football at me and hit me smack on my right nipple. It really hurt, but I didn't want him to know too much about me—he's like 10 years old—so I just pretended it didn't hurt that bad. That was yesterday and my nipple is still sore!

Y'Sheeva, 13

I wonder why my bra sometimes feels a little damp on the inside. Maybe my breasts are sweating or something?

Marisol, 17

I never take my sports bra off in the locker room. Ever! It's not because I have such big breasts. I'm actually kind of flat. It's because my nipples are humongous! My mom said not to worry . . . but she doesn't know how mean people can be. And so far, looking around, I haven't seen another girl with nipples like mine.

Ming, 16

I'm on the swim team and when I first dive into the water, my nipples get really hard. It doesn't hurt, but I feel a little self-conscious when I climb out of the pool.

Megan, 18

First Things First

Nipples are the most prominent parts of your breasts, the part people first notice, often because—much to your embarrassment—they may show right through your clothing. And when you get wet or cold, they scrunch up and stick out even further. In addition, your nipples are usually the most sensitive parts of your breasts, and two of the most

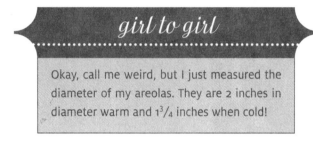

girl to girl

My nipples are psychic: they tell me the future . . . or at least when my period's about to start! A few days before my period, my nips stand up a little bit stiffer and get super-sensitive.

sensitive parts of your entire body. So it's no surprise that nipple issues can take front and center stage in your life.

Here's the Scoop

Nipples and areolas come in a lot of shapes and sizes. Some are large and others are small. Some nipples produce fluid, and some have hair growing from them. Nipples come in a whole spectrum of colors, as we've discussed, from pale pink to dark brown. There is no "normal" type of nipple. Nipples are as unique as you.

girl to girl

Okay, call me weird, but I just measured the diameter of my areolas. They are 2 inches in diameter warm and $1^3/_4$ inches when cold!

Size and Color Combos

There are all sorts of size and color combinations for nipples and areolas. Some nipples can be as long as an inch and as wide as your pinky finger. Some girls have very dark-colored areolas that tend to show through their clothes. Finding bras to conceal big or dark nipples—for "nipple discretion"—is addressed in Chapter 8.

Flat Nipples

Most nipples point out, like an "outie" belly-button. But some nipples are flat or point inward, like an "innie." Nipples like these are called *inverted*. About 10–20 percent of girls have inverted nipples on one or both sides.

Nipples that face inward may eventually change direction and point outward. Even if your nipples stay inverted, they cause no health problems. (Breast-feeding with inverted nipples might be somewhat harder to do, but it is usually manageable.)

Nipple Tips

Do tell a parent or doctor if your nipple once stuck out but then became inverted. It's probably nothing to worry about, but a simple checkup can ensure that everything's okay.

Nipple Fluid

If you notice a small stain in the center of the inside of your bra, it might be fluid that came out of your nipple. Or maybe you were feeling your breasts and you noticed a little drop of nipple fluid. It can happen on one or both sides. Doctors call this *nipple discharge.*

Don't panic! Behind your nipples, inside your breasts, are milk-making glands whose "drainage pipes" all empty out into the openings in the middle of your nipple. (There are more than a dozen of these pipes, also called ducts.) You might be surprised to know that the milk glands are active even without breast feeding. They can make a small amount of fluid—usually clear, slightly yellow, or even milky—which can drain out of the nipple. Occasionally you might even see a little blood that's bright or dark red. This can come from an overgrowth of cells in one of the main milk pipes behind the nipple. Most of the time there's no problem at all. But just to make sure, it's important for your doctor to check things out by testing the fluid.

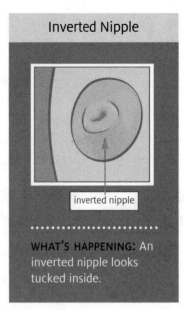

Inverted Nipple

inverted nipple

WHAT'S HAPPENING: An inverted nipple looks tucked inside.

Hair Around Your Nipples and Areolas

Some girls may get hair on or around their areolas or in the middle of their chest between their breasts. Usually it's evenly distributed on both breasts. Most of the time, extra hair, even if unwelcome, is normal. But if you think you have a lot of extra hair, talk to your doctor. You may have an imbalance of hormones that can be corrected.

You can leave the hair alone or you can remove it. Ways to remove unwanted hair are discussed later, in the questions section.

Bumps on Your Areolas

If you have a red, swollen, and tender little bump on your areola, it could be an infection in one of the Montgomery glands. These tiny glands' job is to make a small amount of mucus (so small you can't see it) to keep the nipple and areola soft and moist. If the Montgomery gland gets blocked up, it can get infected, just like a pimple. The good news is that it's pretty easy to treat—particularly if you take care of it quickly.

Don't squeeze or rub it. That will just make it worse. Apply a warm washcloth three times a day followed by an antibiotic ointment, such as Neosporin or Bactroban (available over the counter). Do this for a full week. Your symptoms should improve within a few days and go away completely after a week or so. If the redness and tenderness get worse, see your doctor immediately. It's likely that he or she will want to start a prescription antibiotic medicine right away.

girl to girl

Check out some of the women who walk out of the water on the beach or come out of the shower in a locker room. When you get cold, your nipples *and* areolas shrink up and stick out. Sometimes you can see the Montgomery glands all scrunched up around an erect nipple if it gets cold enough. As soon as you (and your nipples and areolas) warm up, everything relaxes and flattens back down.

Extra Nipples and Breast Tissue

Sometimes even the best design can take unexpected turns. Remember we told you, back in the breast development chapter, that the rest of the mammary ridge disappears when you're an embryo, leaving only two spots, one on each side of your chest, which eventually turn into breasts? Well, every once in a while, a tiny bit of *extra ridge tissue* is left behind. The most common place for an extra nipple to occur is below the left breast. But they can also occur anywhere along the mammary ridge between your armpits and your thighs. The extra ridge tissue can form an extra nipple while you're still in your mom's uterus. As if it wasn't complicated enough getting one set of breasts!

Nipple Tips

But it's good to know that extra nipples are uncommon, and chances are it's something you don't have to worry about. About one to five people out of a hundred have them (1–5 percent). Boys and men are more likely to have extra nipples than girls and women. Most of the time, no one, including you, even notices them. But your doctor might see one and point it out to you. You may even hear your doctor describe them with fancy terms like *accessory breast tissue* or *supernumerary nipples.*

Yeah, having an extra nipple sounds weird—but it's nothing to

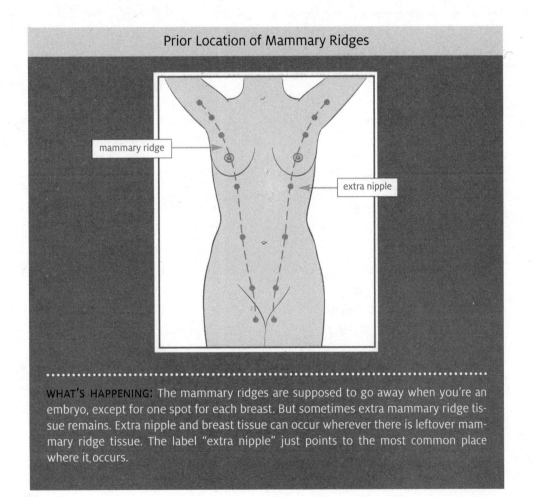

Prior Location of Mammary Ridges

mammary ridge

extra nipple

WHAT'S HAPPENING: The mammary ridges are supposed to go away when you're an embryo, except for one spot for each breast. But sometimes extra mammary ridge tissue remains. Extra nipple and breast tissue can occur wherever there is leftover mammary ridge tissue. The label "extra nipple" just points to the most common place where it occurs.

worry about. If you have extra nipples and breast tissue that make you feel self-conscious, uncomfortable, or embarrassed, share your concern with your parents and your doctor. This extra tissue can be easily removed.

Any Questions?

Is it unusual for your nipples to change from day to day?

When your breasts first start growing, your nipples and areolas can appear big, puffy, and tender almost overnight. It's pretty common for nipples and areolas to change from scrunched up, small, dark, and pointy to flat, lighter, and wider—depending on the temperature and if you're wet or dry, relaxed or tense. When your areolas shrink up, they appear darker and stick out more. All of these changes are completely normal.

Is it bad if your nipples itch?

Your nipples and areolas are full of nerve endings that are very sensitive. If they get brushed the wrong way, bumped, or pinched, *ouch*—they'll immediately let you know they are not happy about it. And when your nipples (and areolas) grow or sense anything new happening underneath, inside the breast, they can feel itchy. These are all normal feelings and nothing to worry about.

How do I get rid of hair on or around my breasts?

Believe it or not, the best way to remove unwanted hair around the areola is with a small pair of scissors. But be careful. To avoid cutting yourself, hold the scissors with your thumb and your first finger, and steady your hand by resting your last two fingers on the surface of your breast.

> ### girl to girl
>
> I have a friend who is a total goofball. She's an actress who is outspoken and loves to make people laugh. She has this funny-looking birthmark on her stomach that she is convinced is an extra nipple. Every time she has a chance to use it as joke material, she does. As long as it makes her and the people around her smile, she doesn't care how embarrassing it could be. She's totally proud of her extra nipple!

Nipple Tips

Plucking the hair with a tweezers is another option, but it might hurt a bit. With this method, the hair won't grow back for several weeks. Laser hair removal is also an option if you have a lot of hair or if you are very troubled by it. Laser hair removal is considered fairly painless, but it is a lot more expensive than the do-it-yourself treatments.

Don't shave—it's too easy to cut yourself since the areola surface is bumpy. The areola skin may also be too sensitive for hair-removal creams and bleaches. And waxing the nipple/areola area—*ouch*—is a definite no-no.

For hair in between your breasts, in the cleavage area, you can wax, shave, use hair removal creams, pluck, or turn to laser removal or electrolysis. When you're trying to figure out which option might work best for you, the people right around you can probably help the most. First, ask some of the women in your family who may have similar hair concerns and share your skin type (dark or fair). They've probably already found a solution that works for them. Your local beauty salon usually has an expert on hair removal. And, your doctor may have some good suggestions.

What do extra nipples/areolas look like?

An extra nipple can look like a dark or pink small bump—sort of like a mole. Sometimes there's both a nipple and an areola, but usually a miniature version. You might also notice a little mound of breast tissue underneath the extra nipple. Together, the extra nipple and mound can look like a tiny extra breast. This extra breast is called an *accessory breast*. Not the kind of accessory you dreamed of pairing with your jeans!

At birth and up until puberty they may be very hard to see. Then with puberty, when your main breasts are growing, the extra nipple (and maybe extra breast tissue) may become noticeable. Sometimes you may not notice an extra nipple until later in your life, during pregnancy.

You can share your stories at TakingCareOfYourGirls.com.

I feel a little bump behind my left nipple and it hurts. But my right one doesn't feel the same way. So I worry that there is something wrong with me.

Lisa, 12

Normal Breast Changes:

Lumps, Cysts, Thick Areas, Pain

We learned in a health class about how our breasts have these glands that produce milk. Some of the girls thought that was gross, but I think it's really amazing! We women have this amazing power.

Amaranta, 16

When my breasts first started developing, it hurt when I'd hug anybody. Once I yelped, "Ouch!" And my friend asked, "What's wrong?" I was so embarrassed! All I could say was "Nothing, nothing."

Madeline, 16

I can predict the arrival of my period depending on how much my breasts hurt. They get big, hard as rocks, and feel like enormous bruises. Sometimes I get what I call the "four-boob effect," when my breasts bubble out over the top of the bra cup and look like a whole other set of breasts.

Claire, 18

When I was thirteen, I worried because my breasts hurt so much—but it was just me starting puberty!

Tawni, 20

I pulled an all-nighter writing a paper for an English class and I drank a ton of coffee! The next day my breasts really hurt. I guess that's a side effect of the caffeine.

Sam, 17

Sometimes my breasts sting and hurt a little. My mom says that's just growing pains.

Angelica, 12

On vacation my cousin was trying to squeeze into the car. She accidentally elbowed my mom in the breast, causing a lump. My mom had the lump removed and it turned out to be nothing.

Margo, 15

I felt a lump in my breast, got really scared, and was so sure I was going to die. My mom took me to the doctor right away. After a bunch of tests, it turned out to be a fibroadenoma. I don't really know what that means, but my doctor told me not to worry about it.

Akeelah, 16

I finally figured out that I have to wear a loose bra at night when I'm about to get my period. Otherwise, I'm lying there in the dark trying not to move at all because it hurts so much!

Melanie, 14

It's really crazy. First our moms and aunts tell us all about breast cancer and how you have to look for lumps and all that stuff. But then they forget to tell us about all the little lumps and bumps that don't have anything to do with cancer at all. They can be just a normal part of getting breasts. How come nobody talks about all this stuff?

Chloe, 15

First Things First

Your breasts are very busy parts of your body. They're not just mounds of fat, and they aren't there just for show—they're glands with a very important job to do: make milk especially designed to nourish human babies. This calls for a pretty complicated dairy system!

From the time you start growing breasts, and for all your life, there's a lot happening on the inside. Along the way, you may notice inside changes, which may make you concerned. This chapter will help you understand and deal with the most common changes inside your "girls."

Here's the Scoop

Your breasts are busy doing all kinds of things inside. When they first start to grow, you might feel a lump in the center of your breast, under your nipple—on one or both sides, of the same or different sizes. These are your breast buds, which give rise to your breast tissue. Even after your breasts develop, part of this pebble-like structure can persist behind your nipples for years, even after your breasts are full-grown.

The development of the milk-making glands is a big construction project. The gland is made up of lobules, where the milk is made, and ducts, which drain the milk. All of these tiny parts work closely together and stay very busy.

The cells that make up these structures normally grow and rest, grow and rest, grow and rest—every day. Your cells' growth and rest periods are controlled by a bunch of different things, but your hormones have the greatest influence.

The main hormones that turn breast cell activity on and off are estrogen and progesterone. When hormone levels go up the breast cells can get excited—causing overactive breast cells or extra breast cell growth. Most of the normal changes you notice on the inside of your breasts are due to this extra activity.

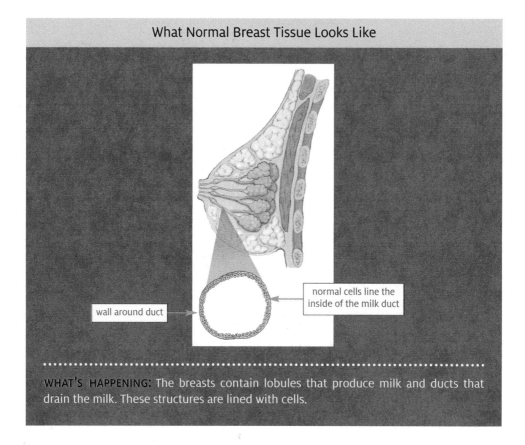

What Normal Breast Tissue Looks Like

wall around duct

normal cells line the inside of the milk duct

WHAT'S HAPPENING: The breasts contain lobules that produce milk and ducts that drain the milk. These structures are lined with cells.

Extra Breast Tissue

Inside breast tissue isn't always smooth and even. Some spots are neat and orderly, and other areas can be lumpy with overactive breast cells or extra breast cells acting out in a number of ways. The extra cells can build up throughout your breasts, making them feel full, firm, stiff, heavy, and even hard. Or there can be extra tissue in a section of the breast, forming an area of thickening (like a scouring pad) or a bumpy region (like a bowl of oatmeal). Or it can build up in one spot, forming a lump that can feel like a grape, a nut, or the tip of your nose. All of these changes can be very confusing.

Normal Breast Changes

Under the microscope, extra breast cell growth may be described as *hyperplasia* (*hyper-* means "too much," *-plasia* means "growth"). If there are extra cells on the inside of a duct, they call it *ductal hyperplasia*. If they are inside the lobule, it's called *lobular hyperplasia*. Most of the time, the extra cells look just like regular breast cells and are perfectly normal. But sometimes the extra cells can look a little unusual under the microscope, in which case they may be described as *atypical* breast cells. These cells will usually stay completely normal but can act up every once

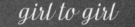
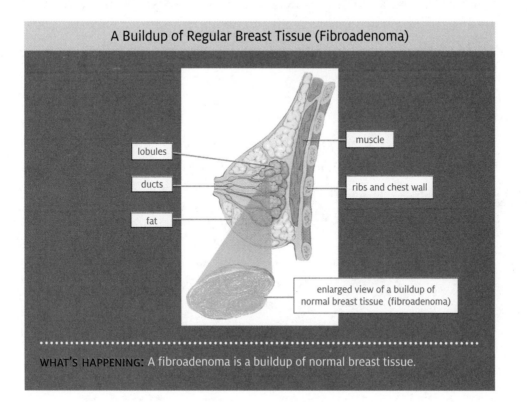

A Buildup of Regular Breast Tissue (Fibroadenoma)

lobules

ducts

fat

muscle

ribs and chest wall

enlarged view of a buildup of normal breast tissue (fibroadenoma)

WHAT'S HAPPENING: A fibroadenoma is a buildup of normal breast tissue.

in a while. This just means your doctor will want to check you over time, particularly if there are breast problems that run in your family.

Sometimes extra breast tissue can roll up or bunch up together, sort of like a ball of yarn or a ball of clay. It can feel like a rubbery, smooth little egg or a tiny football that can be wiggled or moved around within the breast tissue that surrounds it. It's usually painless. Your doctor might say it's a *fibroadenoma*: *fibro-* means "extra scar tissue" and *-adenoma* means "extra gland tissue."

There may be just one in one breast, but sometimes there can be more than one in both breasts. It is not unusual for a fibroadenoma to become tender, particularly prior to the beginning of your menstrual period. This is the most common type of lump in girls between their teens and twenties. Very occasionally, one can get very big, making the breast look bigger than the other side. This is called a *juvenile fibroadenoma* and should be checked out by a breast specialist. Almost always, a fibroadenoma is totally benign. Very, very rarely is breast cancer found in or near a fibroadenoma. If it stays the same size or gets smaller, your doctor will probably tell you to leave it alone.

Cysts

Overactive cells or extra cells can also make extra fluid. Over time, the fluid can fill up and stretch out part of a milk duct, forming a cyst—something like a water balloon.

Some girls have little cysts throughout their breasts, some get just one big cyst, and others get a cluster of cysts in one section of the breast. Any combination of cysts is possible. They may stay the same or change over time, increasing and decreasing in size throughout your menstrual cycle (and driving you crazy).

girl to girl

For as long as I can remember, I've slept on my stomach, but when my breasts got bigger it became too uncomfortable. My weight would squash them on the mattress and it was painful. Finally, I came up with a solution. I still sleep on my stomach, but I move my breasts to the side so they're more comfortable.

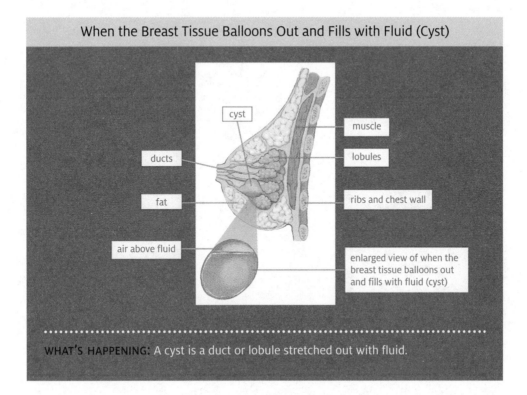

When the Breast Tissue Balloons Out and Fills with Fluid (Cyst)

cyst

muscle

ducts

lobules

fat

ribs and chest wall

air above fluid

enlarged view of when the breast tissue balloons out and fills with fluid (cyst)

WHAT'S HAPPENING: A cyst is a duct or lobule stretched out with fluid.

When fluid builds up inside a cyst and puts pressure on the surrounding breast tissue, it can cause discomfort and pain. Other than this, cysts don't have any negative side effects.

Extra Breast Tissue and Cysts

When there are *both* pockets of extra fluid and extra breast tissue, your doctor might describe this as *fibrocystic breast changes*. The term *fibrosis* comes from extra breast fibers. Your breasts can feel like a lot of little grapes (cysts) throughout a stiff bowl of oatmeal (extra tissue). Not fun, but nothing to worry about.

Both the cysts and the extra breast tissue are very sensitive to hormones. Before your menstrual cycle, when your hormone levels are

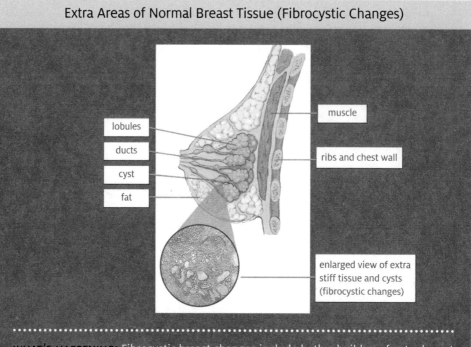

Extra Areas of Normal Breast Tissue (Fibrocystic Changes)

lobules

ducts

cyst

fat

muscle

ribs and chest wall

enlarged view of extra stiff tissue and cysts (fibrocystic changes)

WHAT'S HAPPENING: Fibrocystic breast changes include both a buildup of extra breast tissue and pockets of extra fluid.

super-high, your breasts can get swollen and uncomfortable. Ups and downs of hormone levels at other times of the month can make those changes feel better or worse. How breast tissue reacts to hormones varies a lot from one girl to the next. Fibrocystic changes are basically normal and don't lead to anything serious.

Breast Bumps and Bruises

Getting bumped on the breast can cause a lump or an area of thickening inside. This can happen during athletics, or maybe running into somebody's elbow in the hallway at school. Sometimes you might see a black-and-blue mark on the outside of your breast but you can't remember how it got there.

Normal Breast Changes

Occasionally, a lot of extra upper-body exercise can cause a bruise in the muscle under your breast, making you think you might have a lump in your breast.

Lumps from bumps and bruises are usually due to a buildup of blood or fluid. This usually goes away, but sometimes very slowly. Sometimes scar tissue fills in a bruised area, making it feel firm and hard. Most of the time bumps and bruises disappear without a trace.

Breast Pain, Discomfort, Sensitivity, and Tenderness

Your breasts have many nerve endings that can make them very sensitive to being touched, bumped, or pressured (like lying on your stomach). Your nipples tend to be particularly sensitive because they have the most nerve endings. Plus, many small nerves from the rest of the breast come together near the nipple—that's why feelings from any part of your breast may be felt mostly in your nipple area.

Some girls feel breast discomfort only before their periods, while other girls may feel pain all the time that gets worse at certain times of the month. Once your period starts, the discomfort tends to ease up.

Frustrations and Worries

Many of these normal changes can make examining your breasts difficult

girl to girl

Sometimes I feel like my breasts try on cysts for size! Almost every time before I get my period, I feel a little something new in one or both of my breasts. My mom tells me they're just little cysts that develop because my hormones get all out of whack around my period. Sometimes they're as small as the head of a pin and sometimes they're as big as one of those red-and-white striped mints. I don't like it when my boobs feel weird and bumpy, but the cysts go away after my period. Now, I've just gotten used to my pre-period breasts.

girl to girl

Breasts can get all moody on you. As if my period isn't enough to deal with, my breasts sometimes hurt a few days before it starts. How annoying! They get in my way when I'm already way too busy to deal with it all. Pre-period, I definitely have a love-hate relationship with my breasts.

and at times frightening. The lumps and bumps can feel like grapes, rocks, or pebbles, making you think that something bad might be going on. But don't worry: breast gland tissue normally feels lumpy and bumpy. Lumps can be of different sizes and shapes. Some might feel smooth on the outside like an egg, and others may have a bumpy surface like a corncob or cauliflower. You can usually wiggle the lumps around.

All of these changes might stay the same, go away, or become more noticeable. None of the feelable changes discussed in this chapter—plain hyperplasia, cysts, fibrocystic changes, bumps, and bruises—is associated with a higher risk of breast cancer. Atypical breast cells, described earlier in this chapter, usually don't lead to any problems, but they do have to be monitored by your doctor over the years.

Any Questions?

I'm scared! I have a lump behind my nipple. What do I do?
Take a deep breath! If there is a lump in the center of your breast—one side or both—and if your breasts are still growing, that lump may be part of your breast bud and a necessary part of normal breast development. If you are concerned about the lump, be sure to see a breast care specialist.

Why do my nipples hurt so much?
Your breast is a very sensitive part of your body, and your nipples tend to be particularly sensitive to touch, bumps, or pressure (like lying on your stomach). That's because they have the most nerve endings plus

they're on the surface, stick out the furthest, and are the most likely parts of the breast to get rubbed the wrong way.

How can I make my breasts less lumpy and less painful?

The key to comfort is good breast support. During times of extra breast fullness and pain, support from a full-coverage, well-fitting athletic bra holds you up and in and keeps you comfortable. A looser-fitting nighttime bra can also be helpful.

Heat (or cold) with pressure can help (a hot water bottle can be used with warm or cold water). Try one temperature at a time to see which one works best for you. You can also use a heating pad. Avoid using a very hot temperature so you don't burn yourself.

In general, a balanced diet rich in fruits, vegetables, and grains is recommended.

When it comes to specific foods and drinks, every girl is different. Staying away from caffeine in drinks (coffee, tea, and some soft drinks) and foods (coffee ice cream) may help. Avoiding foods that have caffeine-like substances in them, such as chocolate, might also make a difference. You might also want to avoid salty foods because they may cause you to retain extra fluid, making your breasts feel even fuller.

Some girls notice less breast discomfort after using vitamin E, vitamin B_6, niacin, or herbal products. But don't use any of these without first talking to your doctor.

Your doctor may suggest pain medications to ease discomfort, such as aspirin, acetaminophen, or ibuprofen.

If you experience really bad breast pain that doesn't respond to these remedies and diet changes, your doctor might prescribe medicine to change your hormone levels. Birth control pills are sometimes used for this purpose.

girl to girl

You can feel the different levels of sensitivity of your breasts really easily. Gently roll some of your breast skin between your index finger and thumb. Now do the same thing with your areola and nipple. Feel the difference? Your nipple and areola are so much more sensitive than the rest of your breast. Pretty cool, if you ask me!

I have one cyst that really hurts. What can I do about it?

If you have a lot of pain that you believe is coming from a cyst, have your doctor check it out. Your doctor might order an ultrasound to make sure it's just a straightforward cyst. If it is, removal of the fluid can quickly relieve the pain. This is done with a needle and only takes a few minutes in the doctor's office (don't worry: the needle part is only a quick ouch). After drainage, the cyst might stay deflated or it could eventually fill up again with fluid over weeks to months.

Is a biopsy ever necessary for a cyst?

Simple cysts can be left alone. No biopsy is required (a biopsy is when tissue is removed for examination under a microscope). But if the cyst starts to feel different, then an ultrasound test may be done. And if the test shows a lump or thick areas in the wall of the cyst that persists over time, then a biopsy might be recommended.

How do I know if I have fibrocystic changes?

Fibrocystic changes can often be felt as lumps and bumps in part or all of both breasts. They usually become more noticeable as your period approaches—and often more uncomfortable. If you are concerned, ask your doctor to check out your lumps and bumps at your next visit.

girl to girl

Phew! It's good to know that fibrocystic breast changes aren't a disease, because if they were, I'd have a bad case of it. Before my period, my breasts go nuts. They balloon up and out, requiring a bra that's a whole cup size bigger. As soon as I walk into Mom's office, she knows immediately that I'm about to get my period.

My doctor told me I have fibrocystic breast disease. Is that as bad as it sounds?

Fibrocystic breast changes used to be called a disease. But it's not a disease because it involves normal changes, which are quite common. Plus, fibrocystic changes are not associated with an increased risk of serious problems (such as breast cancer).

Normal Breast Changes

Do I need to be followed extra carefully if I have fibrocystic breast changes?

Fibrocystic breast changes are normal, particularly when your breasts are still growing, but they can persist even into your 30s and beyond. Girls with fibrocystic breasts are followed pretty much the same way as girls with smooth breast tissue.

Check in with your doctor if you feel something that's different from the rest of the surrounding breast tissue and that's not going away or might be getting bigger.

Do I need to be followed extra carefully if I have a fibroadenoma?

Your doctor might want to examine you a few extra times over six months to make sure that everything is stable and on track. An ultrasound might be recommended to check things out further. Occasionally, depending on your age and family history, an MRI scan might be done to get a closer look. A mammogram may be done for a girl in her 20s.

When should a fibroadenoma be removed?

Typical fibroadenomas, which are smooth on the outside and moveable within the breast, are left alone as long as they stay the same size or get smaller. If they get bigger or take on an irregular shape, your doctor will probably want to check things out to make sure that everything is okay and that it's nothing more serious than a fibroadenoma. To check the cells on the inside, a biopsy is usually done. Most commonly it's done with a special needle. Sometimes a biopsy through an incision may be done.

If you or your parents ever doubt a decision to biopsy or remove a fibroadenoma, a second opinion (another doctor's opinion of your case) is a good idea.

What's the best kind of doctor to do a breast procedure on me?

You only want a breast specialist to do any type of breast procedure. An experienced breast surgeon or radiologist knows how to stay away from the nerves of the breast so your breast sensation remains normal, and how to hide an incision so it doesn't show when you wear a bathing suit or tank top. Incisions along the tops of the breasts, particularly in the middle (the area that would show if you were wearing a low-cut tank or bathing suit) tend to show and not disappear very well, so you want to avoid that location whenever possible. Incisions can be easily hidden along the edge of the areola or along the sides or bottom of the breasts. A breast specialist is also most capable of getting a good piece of tissue from the area of concern. Important considerations such as these are the reasons why it's key to see a breast care specialist before deciding on or doing a breast procedure.

You can share your stories at TakingCareOfYourGirls.com.

part two

taking care
of your
"girls"

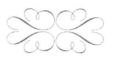

In the fifth grade, I walked by a boy who fake-sneezed and said, "hey, got a tissue?" implying that I stuffed (which I didn't).

Taylor, 16

Self-Image and Teasing:

Standing Up for Yourself and Feeling Your Personal Power

My mom told me I could stuff the top of my dress with some of my brother's socks.

Sara, 12

Once this kid on my bus said that I stuff my bra, when I definitely don't, and I took that personally because I *hate* it when people make fun of me.

Alyssa, 12

A guy told me he wouldn't go out with me because my boobs were too small.

Erin, 15

I was the first person in my grade to get a bra, and I was teased a little for about a day.

Hailey, 10

My friend told me I was flat as a board. She wasn't trying to hurt me, but I felt a little insulted.

Trinity, 11

Lots of times my friend says *my* chest is small, but *hers* is way smaller than mine! She just wears a padded bra to cover it up and then she makes fun of others.

Brooklyn, 16

My friends and I are smaller than most girls our age. One boy was trying to be funny while we were all joking about it at school, and he pointed to our breasts and said, "The only straight As you've got are right there!"

Riley, 14

In seventh grade I got called "Tissues" for no reason. What was worse was that it was my friends who did it to me. I never did use tissues (or anything else) to make my breasts look bigger, yet everyone believed it because of a stupid rumor!

Lily, 18

Someone asked a friend of mine if she would rather trade breast sizes with me (she has pretty big ones). Then my "friend" looked me right in the *eyes* and said, "No way! Why would I ever want to be flat?"

Aaliyah, 12

Guys would stare, as a joke, but it gets annoying and I don't think guys understand it. They think that the attention would be good, but it's embarrassing.

Jenya, 15

I walked by a bunch of boys and they mooed at me to make fun of me.

Mary-Kate, 10

Most of my friends are bigger than me, so they make jokes. They are all Bs and I'm an A. One of them is a C and I'm so jealous!

Jovita, 14

My family jokes around that my breasts are too big because they don't know where they come from, since all my relatives have small ones.

Francesca, 18

My friend was teased with a poem: "Roses are red / Violets are black / Why is your front / As flat as your back?"

Annie, 13

I just laughed off what they said. You can't take yourself or what they say too seriously! When the bully sees you getting upset, they'll keep teasing. If they see that it doesn't bother you, they'll let it go. However, if someone continued to tease me about my breasts, I would take more serious action. I would probably talk to them about it.

Dana, 17

I think it's best to just ignore the teasing. Either they're just jealous or they're insecure with themselves. If you don't have a nasty comeback to say to them, then they will stop teasing you.

Sam, 15

Well, we all grow at a different pace, so what? Maybe you're too big or small. Who is to say what is normal?

Ming, 16

First Things First

"A carpenter's dream." "Torpedo tits." "Tomatoes." "Tissues." "Grapefruit." Did you ever hear of the saying, "Sticks and stones will break my bones, but names will never hurt me"? Unfortunately, it's not that easy to dismiss teasing because it does hurt—sometimes a lot.

Are you being teased about your breast size? You can be a target of hurtful comments, rude remarks, and even harassment, whether you're developing slower than your friends or are way ahead. And sometimes the hurt doesn't go away, even after you've all pretty much evened out size-wise.

Sure, if you're being teased, you feel bad. But remember: *you* are the key to how you feel about yourself, and you have many wonderful qualities. So how do you handle teasing about your breasts? Do you answer back? If so, what do you say? Or do you turn away and say nothing? Will ignoring stop the teasing, make the teaser think you're weak, or make the bad feelings linger?

In this chapter, we'll help you understand why people tease about breasts, how you can handle the teasing, and how you can develop healthy ways to look at your body and appreciate it for what it is. The work it takes to turn off the teasing will empower you. You will feel powerful when you overcome the challenges that come with teasing.

Here's the Scoop

Let's face it: when you start to develop, there's no way to hide it. Your breasts are front and center, changing for everyone to see. Worst of all, you have no control over what's happening to your body. You may be developing faster than everyone else in your circle of friends; on the other hand, you may be the last one to get started.

Either way, breast development is an easy target for teasing. And because breasts are an easy way to compare yourself to other girls, you can become preoccupied with what's going on: *Am I too small? Have I stopped growing? Am I growing too fast?*

You didn't ask for people's attention, and you may not fully understand why you're getting it. There are other pressures too—school, activities, family—and the last thing you need to worry about is what other people are thinking or saying about your developing breasts and how they should look.

As you develop into a young woman, remember that it's normal to be self-conscious about your body. But also try to remember that you are more than the sum of your two breasts. And what you're experiencing and feeling now is temporary. Your body will continue to change throughout your life. The very things you worry about now may be just the right fit in a year or two.

Who Is Doing the Teasing?

People can say mean things—even the people you care about. You may be surprised at who teases you about your breasts. It's not always the "idiot boy" with the nasty comment. It can be your best friend, or even your mother or your sister. Even if they never meant to be mean, their comments can hurt just the same—or even more—because it's so *personal* and they're supposed to support you, not bring you down.

There are important differences between a friend saying something thoughtless that hurts your feelings, a flirtatious boy who slips and says something that really bothers you by accident, a family member or close friend who pokes fun at you, or a kid in school who teases you. It's very important to stop the teasing from the people close to you first. You can't feel the comfort, confidence, and strength you need if your loved ones are sending mixed messages to you and about you through teasing. It's hard enough to deal with the teasing on your own, but without your family's support, self-doubt can creep in and take the wind out of your sails just when you need to get out of the storm.

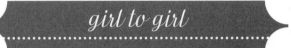

girl to girl

In my close group of friends, we all have different sizes and shapes of breasts. The good thing is that we are all very happy with our respective sizes, big and small. Because we all know this, we're okay with teasing each other about our breast sizes. This kind of teasing is a testament to our trust because we all have confidence that our intentions are not mean. Plus we give just as many compliments to one another as we do playful jabs.

What's Going On in the Teaser's Mind?

Human beings are very complicated. Mean people can be nice and nice people can be mean. How confusing—and how hard to understand it all and keep it straight.

girl to girl

I was called "gorilla legs" on the school bus by a boy who lives in my neighborhood. Turns out kids had been calling him "gorilla legs" because his legs were so hairy. And there I was at age eight—lucky me—on the school bus, wearing shorts with my hairy legs showing. I hadn't even noticed my leg hair, so I had him to thank for bringing it up for the first time. Well, I came home from school sobbing, horrified and embarrassed. My mom called his mother, and that's how we found out that other kids had been teasing him. He never said anything else to me ever again, but I can tell you that the hurt went deep and stuck for a long time.

But one thing is clear: teasing has little to do with you and much more to do with the teaser. It's definitely not your fault. People who tease have often been teased a lot themselves, teaching them by example to tease others and expect to be teased. They are in the bad habit of thinking and feeling bad things about themselves, and if someone else is around, they take the opportunity to make that other person feel bad. Their negative thoughts and feelings can pollute their interactions with other people.

Why Do They Pick on You and Not Someone Else?

You've probably wondered: of all people, why are you the target of someone's mean words? Teasers will pick people they think they can make feel bad quickly and easily. Stopping the teasing means not being the target or the victim. Teasers are also looking for something that's easy to tease someone about. Anything that stands out—like differences between people or something unusual—will grab the teaser's attention right away. Very big breasts, very small breasts, a colored bra under a see-through shirt, or a T-shirt with a clever phrase over the breast area are all potential triggers.

There are a lot of reasons for teasing, but there are a couple of common themes. All seem to come from how others handle anxiety and other complicated feelings.

Girls can tease you because they are anxious, nervous, jealous, or trying to get you to be like them. If you're developing ahead of other girls, they may just be nervous. The difference between their situation and yours raises questions and conflicting feelings for them: *When will my breasts start to grow? Am I too big or too small? When will I need a bra?* By striking first with a tease, they reveal their own insecurity about this sensitive time. Or other girls may be envious. Their teasing lets you know that you're not like them. But they may just want to be where you are.

Friends tease friends to reinforce the way they expect each other to behave. If your breasts are larger than those of your friends and you flaunt it, your friends may tease you to let you know they think you're out of line.

girl to girl

I've endured enough teasing for a couple of lifetimes. Living with two brothers and two more male cousins during the summer has made my skin thick and tough. I've been teased for everything from wanting to take a dance class to the size of my feet (I'm a size 11 wide). My height, my weight, my clothes—you name it, my brothers have probably hassled me about it. Sometimes it's more bearable than other times, but I've learned that the best way to deal with it—to spare yourself some embarrassment and preserve your dignity—is to respond from a position of power.

Your parents or other family members can feel very uncomfortable with the idea of you growing up and becoming a woman. They may say negative things about the very changes, such as your breasts, that *they're* uncomfortable with, making you feel like a child again.

Boys who tease girls about their breasts are showing just how immature they are. Chalk their teasing up to the fact that girls usually mature faster than boys, both physically and mentally.

Teasing can also occur because we're not very good at talking about sexuality or about our bodies in ways other than joking. And if you ask people why they tease, they'll usually say they're just joking. Humor is an easy, familiar, and comfortable way to bring up difficult topics.

No matter what the reasons are for being teased, you don't have to accept it. And we're going to help you figure out what to do to avoid, manage, and overcome being teased.

Teasers are like hungry animals looking for something to eat. Anything less than perfection or anything different looks like food to them. Their idea of "regular," "normal," and "perfect" is not from reality. It probably comes from television, the movies, the Internet, and the covers of magazines. But look around you. How much perfection do you really see? There is no "perfect" or "right" size breast; there is no "normal" size for any particular age, height, or weight. It's totally ridiculous to think everyone should fit one idea of perfection.

What Do You Think?

When someone picks on you, naturally it makes you upset. But if you show your feelings to the teaser, *bingo*—you've just given that person exactly what he or she wants. It will be your ability to think on your feet at the very moment when you're experiencing a mix of hurt and embarrassed feelings that is going to get you through and beyond the teasing encounter.

The key to stopping the teasing is to hold back your emotional reaction, then reflect and think up the best way to respond. The goal is to get you through and beyond the situation feeling whole, empowered, and good about yourself. As hard as it may seem, it is absolutely possible for you to handle these tough situations. Getting through a situation where you're being teased is a skill you def-

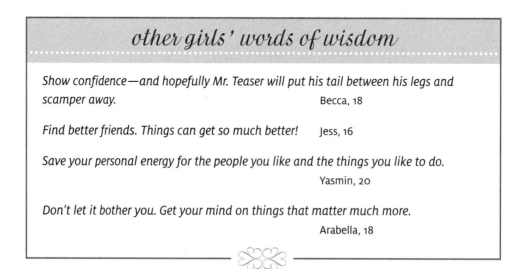

other girls' words of wisdom

Show confidence—and hopefully Mr. Teaser will put his tail between his legs and scamper away.　　　　　　　　　　　　　　Becca, 18

Find better friends. Things can get so much better!　　Jess, 16

Save your personal energy for the people you like and the things you like to do.　　　　　　　　　　　　　　Yasmin, 20

Don't let it bother you. Get your mind on things that matter much more.　　　　　　　　　　　　　　Arabella, 18

initely can master. But like shooting hoops or sewing a shirt or reading French, it requires practice.

Your Own Mental Housekeeping

Before you can effectively deal with people teasing you, you have to start with what's in your own head. Do you have piles of self-doubt cluttering your thinking? Are you unhappy with your body? Are you checking out your breasts on a daily basis, praying for them to be something different? Do you become paralyzed whenever anyone says anything critical, rude, or teasing? Do you refuse to believe a compliment from a friend?

If this is you, we have to work on changing those thoughts immediately. You want to avoid the mind-set of being a victim, now and at any other point of your life. Negative feelings about yourself can leak out, sending cues to other people that you're not in charge and are vulnerable to attacks such as teasing.

You already know what we're going to say: you have to get to work on shifting your way of thinking and feeling from negative to positive, from paralyzed to in charge. An important part of every chapter in this book is about how to get comfortable with yourself, enjoy who you are, and celebrate your uniqueness. Here we want you to focus on all the special things about yourself.

You can use positive self-talk. That's when you remind yourself of your strengths and special gifts and reassure yourself that while no one is perfect, there's nothing wrong with you. It might be helpful to think about why people tease: because they don't have a grip on their own problems ("I'm flunking algebra and she's getting an A"), or they don't understand their own feelings ("I like her, but what if she doesn't like me?"), or they just don't know any better ("My mom makes fun of her sister, so it must be okay"). Understanding where the teaser is coming from is not the same thing as accepting the teasing. If the teaser's words are mean and critical and if you believe that what he or she is saying is true, then it will be impossible for you to come out of the situation feeling empowered or good about yourself.

Teasing from the Home Front and Close Friends

Even after you "clean house" and eliminate your own negative thinking habits, you might also have to address negative feelings coming from your family and close friends. As we've noted, teasing from people close to you deserves a different solution than teasing from others. You need your immediate support network to back you up, not knock you down, and help you gain enough confidence to deal with teasing from the outside world.

When you're teased about your breasts, how does it make you feel? This is important, because how you feel tells you whether you can let the teasing go or if you should respond in some way. If the teasing is annoying but not such a big deal, you can ask the person who's teasing you to stop. Say, "What you're saying bothers me. I'd like you to stop." But if the teasing happens more often and it's bringing you down, then a heart-to-heart talk is needed. Here, asking questions can help start the conversation and make the person close to you reflect on what he or she is doing or saying. For example, if your mother suggests that you stuff your bra with your brother's socks (like in the quote at the beginning of this chapter), you can say: "Mom, are you disappointed in my breast size and that's why you're telling me to do something like stuff my bra? Because if that's the message that you want to give me, it hurts my feelings as well as my self-image." Or you can say, "Why would you say that to me? You know that the most important thing I need is to feel good about the way I am and the way I look. Without your support and confidence, how am I supposed to handle rude comments and teasing from strangers?"

Responding to an insensitive comment from someone close to you (which reveals *their* insecurity) with a straightforward, honest statement is very powerful. Speaking frankly about your feelings can be really meaningful. And it can show the offender that his or her offhand comment said more to you than he or she intended.

Among friends, there's a level of teasing that's okay—and it might even be a way for you to bond with each other at this sensitive time. If you're developing faster than everyone else, for example, you might jokingly acknowledge that your boobs are pretty big, and you don't take offense if your close friends say something similar. Joking and sharing your feelings can help you sort out the mixed emotions this time of life brings. The easy familiarity you have with each other means you can support each other through the rocky times.

But teasing is not okay if it makes you feel bad and keeps you from feeling good about yourself. Only you can decide when and how to react, and how to behave toward anyone who teases you.

> ## girl to girl
>
> The line between acceptable teasing and unacceptable teasing gets even thinner when it's with friends. I once told a friend that I was self-conscious about my upper arms. A few days later, she made some offhand comment about them. She didn't have malicious intentions, but it didn't feel right when it came out of her mouth, even though I had said it about myself.

Teasing from People You Don't Know So Well

If you're being teased by someone at school, from the neighborhood, or elsewhere and you want it to stop, try the techniques described below.

• **PUSH THE PAUSE BUTTON ON YOUR EMOTIONS.** In response to being teased, the teaser is expecting you to become angry, hurt, confused, and defensive. You don't want to give him or her what he or she wants. Yes, your emotional reaction is immediate and can feel like it's

girl to girl

I've tried every trick in the book when it comes to teasing. I've found that saying something mean or sly back never makes the situation better, and it often makes it worse. I'm not so great at thinking of something witty on the spot, and when I used to try, I'd often just make a bigger fool of myself. I get a good laugh out of those situations now, but it wasn't so great back then.

bursting out of you. Hold your reaction and keep your feelings inside for the moment. Instead, respond in an unexpected way with words the teaser is unable to react to (we'll give you some ideas a little later in this section). Your goal: take care of yourself and get out of the situation.

• REGAIN POWER WITH A POSITIVE RESPONSE. Teasers' minds are full of negative thoughts. So if you respond with a positive thought—such as agreeing with them or complimenting them—it will throw them off balance and make them go away. Agreeing with comments takes their power away. Focus only on something positive in what they say—even if it is just a word and ignore the mean stuff.

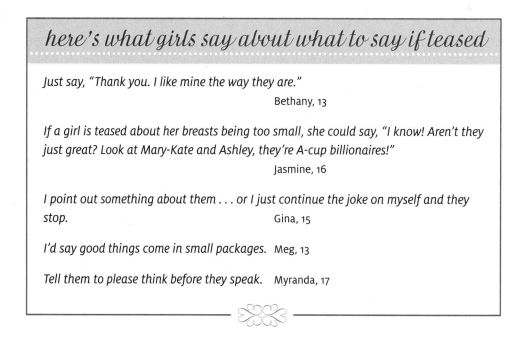

here's what girls say about what to say if teased

Just say, "Thank you. I like mine the way they are."
Bethany, 13

If a girl is teased about her breasts being too small, she could say, "I know! Aren't they just great? Look at Mary-Kate and Ashley, they're A-cup billionaires!"
Jasmine, 16

I point out something about them . . . or I just continue the joke on myself and they stop. Gina, 15

I'd say good things come in small packages. Meg, 13

Tell them to please think before they speak. Myranda, 17

Weave the positive word or thought into your response. For example, if a teaser says: "Ooooh, look, your titties are sooooooo small!" then you can say, "Yes, thanks so much for noticing. They really are the best. Lucky me!" Pause, stand up straight, smile, then walk away and feel your power. Act sincere, like you mean it, and keep your tone of voice thoughtful and sincere. Do not be sarcastic or defensive. Look right at them, establish eye contact, smile, then move on. Keeping control over your body language and tone are essential to the success of your response. Think of yourself as an actress and of this as a play called *Killing Them with Kindness*. But no overacting—act like you mean it.

Responding with these strategies takes time, self-control, and practice. You can practice with your best friend or a family member. Once you try it out a few times, you'll come to understand why and how it will work, you'll gain some confidence, and you'll be ready for any kind of uncomfortable situation.

When Do You Ignore the Remark and Walk Away?

"Ignore it and walk away" is probably the most common advice you'll get from others. This strategy certainly works better than looking defeated, getting upset, or becoming defensive. But teasers expect that you might choose to ignore them. They might give up on teasing if you walk away, since they get little satisfaction, yet it's also possible that they will be tempted to try teasing you again—and maybe push you a little harder—to get the emotional reaction they're seeking.

girl to girl

I've heard my teachers say that visible differences between people are triggers for teasing. Well, I have two brothers and several male cousins whom I live with a lot of the time. When you're the only girl and you're going through puberty, everything about you is different, noticeable, and ripe for their commentary. For them, I am live entertainment. Teasing in my family is definitely a big part of our rivalries, and it's sort of like a game. Sometimes the things we tease each other about are so trivial that what we're really making fun of is the fact that it's so silly.

Ignoring teasing can help you escape the immediate situation, but it doesn't really take care of your feelings. You are unlikely to feel the personal power of overcoming the encounter—and as a result, you might still feel bad, and the teaser might come back for more.

You can consider the source—an immature boy, for example—and ignore it. You can refuse to take the bait and walk away, giving off the attitude that the remark is not worth your time. Or if it's a day when you feel unable to come up with a thoughtful response, ignoring the person is easier, faster, and more effective than letting a flood of emotion burst out. That's more than okay. If there is a next time, it's an opportunity to try again.

What Not to Say

Letting your emotions take over doesn't work. When you feel your emotions rise and they're on the verge of spilling out, reach for the faucet and turn off the flow of feelings. Bottom line: don't get upset in front of the teaser. Other big things to avoid:

- Don't scold or threaten. Never say, "You *should*" anything. Your words will just remind the teaser of useless discipline warnings through the years. Telling the teaser that you'll report him or her or tell your mother is unlikely to change his or her behavior.

- Don't criticize the teaser. Saying things like "You really are a jerk and a stupid, terrible, thoughtless person" will only make things worse.

- Don't give advice or deliver a lecture on how people should be nice to each other and that you expect that he or she will be nice to you. The teaser has heard those lectures a million times before, and your rules and values mean nothing to him or her. As valid as your message might be, it's not going to have any impact on the teaser.

- Don't insult, humor, or make fun of the person. Saying things like "Oh, you think my breasts are small? Well, I heard that your penis is the size of a peanut!" won't give you the result that you're really seeking.

- Don't be defensive. Act from a position of strength. This might require some practice, since the natural response to any kind of attack *is* to be defensive.

- Don't seek revenge or plan a counterattack. This just makes the situation worse, invites more hurtful teasing, causes you anxiety, and gives you no real power. If you get caught up in planning attacks and counterattacks, then things can turn into a mini-war. This approach is nothing but trouble, leading to a downward spiral with a bad outcome.

Remember, your goal is to take care of yourself and get out of the immediate situation. Teaching the teaser a lesson and turning him or her into a better person is *not* a realistic goal (and it's not your job—that's something for the teaser's parents).

The teasing game is one that you have to play as directly as you possibly can. Using substitutes, like a parent or friend, doesn't work as well. But you can definitely use your family and friends for backup and support.

If the teasing gets worse, if you feel bullied or harassed, then you need to bring in people to help you manage the situation. Don't keep the teasing a secret! Teasing can be like a virus. The teaser might step up his or her attacks on you and choose other people to pick on. When you bring in other people such as guidance counselors at school, teachers, the principal, and parents, you can help stop the virus and make the situation better for everyone.

girl to girl

Sometimes you can do a great job with a comeback, but sometimes it can really bomb. Teasing can come at the worst time, when everything is terrible: maybe your parents had a big fight last night, you were late to school, you have a huge zit on your forehead, you have your period, you had a falling-out with your best friend only yesterday, and you forgot your homework. You thought nothing more could possibly happen, and then this total jerk says something mean and stupid. Out comes a flood of tears. Stand back. Everyone is going to get wet. How can you manage getting teased under these circumstances? Maybe not as well—but when the going gets tough, the tough get going! How's this for a try: "Thanks for your comment. I'm so sorry to get so upset on you. Don't worry, it's got nothing to do with you. It's not your fault. Today is a bad day. I could really use someone to talk to. Do you have about an hour?" Stand back and give the guy a little space because he's going to take off like a rocket.

When Teasing Goes Too Far

Teasing goes too far when it hurts you, when it makes you feel uncomfortable. There's no definition you can look up to help you understand the difference between teasing you're willing to accept and teasing that hurts you. There's a very fine line between the two that is easily crossed or misunderstood. Everyone is different, and what bothers you might not bother your best friend. You might be able to brush off teasing about a haircut—after all, hair always grows back. But there's nothing you can do to make your breasts start or stop growing, and teasing about them invades your privacy and hits a sore spot.

Your comfort zone regarding teasing can vary from situation to situation and from one type of teaser to another. But remember, only you can decide. And you're not being wishy-washy. Talking about your breasts is a very delicate thing, and it's not uncommon to go from having a normal conversation to feeling uncomfortable very quickly.

In contrast, if the teasing becomes so serious that you feel bullied or harassed, additional steps need to be taken. Don't handle it alone—reach out for help. You can read more about bullying in the Q&A section.

The Power Lies in You

A huge part of growing up is learning how to stand up for yourself and respond to all different kinds of people at different times under different circumstances. And there will be major lessons and missteps along the way! One of the greatest pleasures life has to offer is rising to face challenges big and small and overcoming them. But there will also be setbacks along the way.

Plenty of times you might want to kick yourself for saying the wrong thing, or second-guess yourself and come up with better things you could have said. Expect that some challenges might turn out differently than you could have imagined. Some will go okay, some won't go so well, and others will feel like major victories—better than winning the Olympics.

But this really is what life is about: ups and downs, and figuring out the best way to deal with both. When things bomb out, see it as a lesson to learn from, not as a mistake. It really is true: all challenges are opportunities to learn about yourself, others, and the world out there—not just teasing challenges.

In the beginning, saying something positive to someone who is being negative might not make any sense to you. But once you practice it and then try it in a few different situations, you'll find that it works quite well. You'll learn how to adapt your approach to new and different situations. With experience, your confidence will build, you will be teased less often, and when you do get teased, you will be able to handle it much better.

Any Questions?

What can I do to stop the teasing before it starts?
There's no guaranteed way to prevent people from teasing you. Some people will say what they want to say even if, or sometimes because, it hurts you. Showing confidence, staying busy doing what you like to do, and having good friends are all ways to reduce the risk that you'll be teased.

Sometimes it helps to know that teasing is a normal part of growing up. If you've just started to develop or are a late bloomer, remember that teasing about your breast size can happen, and people do it for different reasons. The same people who might have picked on a kid's hair or clothes in grade school may now be making boob jokes.

If my friends tease me, does it mean that they're not my friends anymore?
Friends say things to friends that can come out the wrong way and were never meant to be hurtful. For example, let's say you're talking with friends when the conversation turns to your changing bodies and you say something like "I'm waiting for mine to grow." It sounds like you're putting yourself down, so your friends assume that it's okay to tease you. Or your comment makes them notice your barely growing breasts for the first time, giving them a new opportunity to tease you.

What do I do when my friend blabs?

You've just learned something important: this "friend" has broken your trust. Consider telling this friend how hurt you were by her actions, and that she lost your trust. If you feel it's worth it, let the relationship heal and try to rebuild trust. But sometimes that's not possible, no matter how much you try. Your friend might be lots of fun, have great taste in clothes, be good to go shopping with, and be smart and interesting, but exchanging personal information might not be something you should do in this relationship.

You don't want to be too careful or too unforgiving, either—otherwise you might find that you don't want to talk to anyone. That's not a good outcome. People are not perfect—not you, not anyone else.

The next time you tell any of your friends something you don't want other people to know, make that clear to them—or else they might not take you as seriously as you want them to. Tell them straight up: "This is between you and me. I don't want other people to know."

girl to girl

Let's face it: girls love to talk. This can be both a good thing and a bad thing. Especially in middle and high school, things can go badly. There is a whole lot of negative pressure that can make a friend spill a secret intended to stay between you and her. I think we've all found ourselves in situations where it would be easy to slip up. It's important to be wary of these pressures, but don't let it hold you back from creating a bond with someone. I have a few very close girlfriends, and I don't share personal information with many other people.

If a boy teases me, does that automatically mean he's a jerk? What if I still like him?

Puberty is such a tough time for everyone. Your body and your feelings change from day to day. Having a crush on a guy is totally natural, but talking to him can feel very uncomfortable. Sometimes teasing happens almost by accident. Let's say you're talking with a boy you like about things you have in common, and there's some flirting going on. The next thing you know, he's made a comment about your breasts that really upsets you. What went wrong? Why did he stop being cute and charming and funny and start acting like a jerk? In the middle of this awkwardness, you can say the wrong thing and so can he.

When does teasing cross the line and become harassment?
Here's what the law says is harassment: conduct you don't want that violates your dignity or creates a hostile, degrading, or intimidating environment for you. That's a pretty broad definition, but the important thing to know about harassment is that the law also says it's what you feel that counts. In these serious cases, you may have to enlist the help of an adult you trust—your parent, a teacher, a coach, a counselor, or a clergy member. All schools take harassment seriously and have rules against such behavior and guidelines in place for dealing with people who do it.

Two more important things to remember: If you feel you're being bullied, don't keep it to yourself—and don't blame yourself. It's not your fault. No one deserves to be bullied, whether it's about breast size or something else. Reach out to your parent and a school counselor. Don't keep it a secret! And if you're a witness to bullying, don't join in on the bullying; rather, offer support to the person being bullied. That may actually stop it. When you stand up for yourself or for a friend, you can experience a wonderful feeling because you've done the right thing about something that's important. Your connection to your inner feelings gets stronger and the bond with your friends gets tighter. Everyone respects you when you do what's right and show that you care. Of course, all of this takes a lot of courage, but we know that you have it inside you.

It's frustrating trying to talk to my mom. What do I do?
It's not going to be easy all the time. In fact, you'll encounter a bunch of conversation-stoppers and disappointments. Things can come out wrong. Best intentions can land flat, feelings can be hurt, and each of you can miss what the other is saying. Sometimes, just when you managed to get out what you wanted to say, the other person jumps in,

misinterprets what you've said, and launches in on a useless lecture. Even adults can half-listen, interrupt, or hijack the conversation, whether it's intentional or not. When these things happen, it can hurt your feelings, frustrate you, and make you less likely to try again. But don't give up! There's a lot you can learn from each of these situations. Find a time and place to bring up your frustration, and figure out what you want to say beforehand. You don't want to rush this kind of conversation, so allow plenty of time for it. In a calm, private environment free of distractions, talk to this person and tell him or her how you feel. Without being accusative, emphasize to the adult that you're not getting the information you're looking for. Then maybe the two of you can come up with a code word to use when you feel that things are going off track or when she or he is not listening: "Hello!" Or when the conversation is being hogged: "My turn!"

I don't think my mom understands how I feel because she always automatically reassures me. How can I talk to her?
There are times when you may not think you have much in common with your mother, but chances are she knows exactly how teasing feels because she's been there. Sure, it was a long time ago, but teasing about breasts is really not new and it's something no one forgets easily.

Even if your mom has gone through similar stuff, breast development might be an awkward subject to talk about. She may think your breast size is fine, regardless of what you think. You may have to be persistent if you want to talk to her about what's bothering you.

Why do I feel jealous of people I like? It makes me feel bad.
First of all, feeling jealous about people you like is normal. Let's say you're best friends with Laura. But Laura is developing a lot faster than you are, and you're starting to get anxious. As she continues to leave you behind, your anxiety turns to jealousy. Why Laura and not you? Your feelings are natural. But uncontrolled jealousy can damage or even ruin friendships. And it may indicate something about you rather than about the people of whom you are jealous. Do you feel insecure about

your own development? Try to be honest with yourself about why you're jealous. Don't hide from it. If you confront it head-on, you'll have a better chance of overcoming it.

What can be done to stop a rumor about my breasts?

A rumor about your breasts can make you upset or depressed and make you not want to go to school or hang out with your friends. It's hard to face everyone when they believe something about you that isn't true—for example, that you stuff your bra with tissues. Try to find out who started the rumor and ask him or her to stop. Or if you don't want to confront the person directly, ask a friend to stick up for you. Whenever someone brings up the rumor, ask your friend to intervene and tell the truth. And finally, try not to let it continue to upset you. Getting upset is exactly the reaction that people who start rumors want. If you can shrug it off, the person who started the rumor might move on to something or someone else.

How do I deal with Internet teasing?

With today's instant messaging, Facebook, MySpace, text messaging, and e-mail, you may have to contend with more than just words said to your face. The Internet makes you vulnerable to teasing in all sorts of ways your parents never had to worry about. And cyberteasing has one main difference from the hurtful comment said to your face: you have no control over what others are posting about you or who else sees the remarks. A cybertease can take on a life of its own. Teens do it to other teens, and sometimes parents can do it to teens as well.

If you're being teased online, print out the conversation. People can deny a remark; they can't deny anything they put online if you have a copy. If you know the teaser, the best thing to do is confront him or her in a quiet, safe place. While maintaining control of your emotions, tell the person that you know about their teasing and you want it to stop. If they deny it, show them the printout and tell them you will bring it to a parent or a principal if it doesn't stop. Bullies usually have more than one victim, so when you stand up for yourself, chances are you're standing up for other (and future) targets.

You can share your stories at TakingCareOfYourGirls.com.

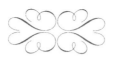

I got one of those Old Navy sports bras and wore it to school. I felt so embarrassed and uncomfortable that I went to the bathroom, took it off, and kept it in my pocket for the rest of the day.

Anjali, 10

Bras for You:

Cami, Athletic, Underwire, Padded, Lace

8

My friend and I had this secret code. Whenever we knew one of our friends was wearing a bra we would make this funny face and laugh about it—but that was then. As we grew up, doing our secret code became more and more uncomfortable because it became clear that we too needed bras. It was hard to admit this to each other.

Lena, 14

I've tried a bunch of times to talk about the fact that—hello, people!—I could really use a bra, but no one seems to listen, care, or know what to say.

Sasha, 11

When I bought my first bra I had to be measured. The woman measured me in front of everyone—and everyone was watching. I was sooooo embarrassed.

Kari, 11

Finding a bra was a real scene. Bigger-sized bras, they're hideous. You can find them in my size in department stores, but they're in the full-figure section, and they're usually really ugly and they have really big straps in the back. Everybody *else* has cute little Victoria's Secret bras or a training bra, and I've got this, like, boulder holder.

Rose, 19

My dad went to the store to buy me my first bra. He had no idea what he was doing, so he just bought *everything* that he thought might fit me. When he got home he put them on my bed and told me to try them on with my mom. My mom ended up having to return all but one bra.

Grace, 12

I got my first bra as a hand-me-down, so no family members even knew. So I was fine!

Madeleine, 12

My mom just bought my little sister fake little training bras, and she is only six. I am overprotective of my sister. So I stole them all so she wouldn't wear them until she got older.

Ashley, 15

I wish I could wear a cup bra, but I'm too small for them. Once I tried one on with a dress and my boobs looked bigger—but I didn't like how it looked. I felt uncomfortable because it wasn't me; it was artificial. If Saturday I was flat-chested and Sunday I showed up to a party with big boobs, what would people say? It would be ridiculous.

Siri, 17

I was out shopping for my first bra with my mother. My mom went up to a *guy* in the store and asked if *he* could help us find a size for me. Turns out the man didn't even work there!

Maryanne, 13

Bras for You

I want a bra to smooth everything out, to flatten the nipple puffiness so it's not noticeable.

Jen, 10

When I got my first bra, my sister referred to it as mosquito netting for the bites.

Molly, 11

My secret advice to my mom: "Gently persist when you want to talk to me about buying a bra, until I give in and listen. (I know it's hard.) Get me in the car. Take me to a store. Just buy it."

Lena, 14

I am rather sensitive and modest, so I was totally humiliated when my mother started to fiddle with the straps of my new bra in front of my father.

Julia, 12

My mother bought me my first bra and said I had to wear it because I was starting junior high school. I didn't really need a bra and the first thing I did every day when I got home was take the darn thing off.

Liz, 19

I first asked for a bra when I was 11 and everyone else was getting one. I absolutely did not need it physically, and when I asked for it, my mother said, "Why would you want that? You don't need it." While she meant well, it was very upsetting to me, and in protest, I basically refused to wear a bra until I was 16, which is when I got my first one.

Jamaica, 18

I did not need a bra, but the girls at school were torturing me. When my mom brought me to buy my first one, the saleslady said very loudly that I didn't need one, so my mom kicked her gently in the leg and then the lady quickly announced loudly, "Oh, you're right, the *training* bras are right over there."

Rayna, 16

My mom gave me a bra ahead of time, saying, "Just in case, for whatever happens, use it now or later." Getting the bra ahead of time made me feel better because it saved me from having to think about getting one—and when the time came for needing it, I had what I needed.

Sasha, 19

A few years ago I had been wearing a 36D, but a bra fitter said, "It's all wrong. It's standing away from your body." She measured me: 34DD. She said the bra should be sitting against your chest, flat. I tried on the 34DD, it fit perfectly, and it was like all of a sudden this lightbulb went on!

Susan, 19

I prefer sports bras because they make me look flatter. Having a grown-up bra makes me feel grown-up, but I'm too scared to switch. Besides, my boobs don't seem to fill in the cups. I don't want the bra or my nipples showing through a shirt, and I don't want my family—particularly my brothers—to see and make comments.

Lena, 14

First Things First

The whole idea of a bra started about 6,500 years ago in Greece. Women wore this very odd thingamajig for breast support during exercise. It held up their breasts, but it didn't cover their nipples. The women did sports with their breasts showing!

Shooting a bit forward in bra history, Henry S. Lesher of Brooklyn, New York, invented a sort of bra in 1859 designed to give a "symmetrical rotundity." The woman in this picture doesn't look too happy, does she?

A more modern bra was patented in 1914 by a woman named Mary Phelps Jacob. She marketed her bras under the name Caresse Crosby (don't ask us who Crosby was, 'cause we don't know ☺). Her bra was made of two silk handkerchiefs with baby ribbon straps. She sold the patent to the Warner Brothers Corset Company for $1,500!

The year 1977 marked another milestone in bra history. Runners Hinda Miller and Lisa Lindahl created the Jogbra, the first sports bra, by stitching two jock straps together. Since then, exercise bras have come a long way and offer levels of support for different types of physical activity.

For thousands of years, women have depended on bras for real support, coverage, comfort, and style so they can lead their fun and full lives. Now there are so many choices, it can be hard to know how to pick the right bra for you. Read on for some good advice.

Here's the Scoop

Your breasts are very sensitive, delicate parts of your body and need help to stay protected, and that's where a bra comes in handy. A bra's two main jobs are to give your breasts support and to cover your breasts so you feel more comfortable in clothes. No matter what your size—small, medium, large, extra-large—your breasts need support as you walk, run, dance, or flip.

Other parts of your body, such as your head, arms, and legs, have bones inside to give them strength and support. But your breasts have no bones. The skin provides some support on the outside, but most of their support comes from an inner network of tiny threads, called Cooper's ligaments, which act like inside shock absorbers for your breasts. But these ligaments are also fragile, and they too need support to keep from stretching out. If they get stretched, they are less able to absorb all the bounces, twists, and turns that happen as you move around. Over time and without proper support, your breasts can sag. The bigger your breasts are, the lower their position will be. Plus, bouncing breasts hurt. A good bra that holds your breasts in place actually makes you much more comfortable as you do all the activities that you want to do.

But for a bra to work for you, it has to fit right. And, as it turns out, most girls and women are walking around wearing the wrong size bra.

Parts of a Bra

There are three main parts of a standard bra that are designed to give support: the band, the cups, and the straps. The bra band goes around your chest underneath your breasts and is supposed to support most of the weight of your breasts. The bra's cups hold your breasts up in position and shape how they look under your clothes. Finally, the straps connect the top of the cups to the back of the band.

Figuring Your Bra Size Yourself

Band and Cup Size

Measure yourself to get a rough idea of your size. (Later on, when you're ready to buy a bra, work with a bra fitter in the store to get a more accurate reading.)

To get started, all you need is a tape measure and a private place. If it's your first bra, you can measure with nothing on or over a thin shirt.

Bras for You

If you already have a bra that you think fits pretty well, you can measure over it (as long as it's unpadded and not too tight).

Bra size is based on two things: band size (a number) and cup size (a letter)—for example, 36C. To get your bra band size, measure all the way around your rib cage, right under your breasts. Make sure the tape measure goes straight around your body, parallel to the floor. Keep the measuring tape flat against your body—don't let it dig in, twist, or ride up your back. Now it gets a bit more complicated. Round out the number up or down to the nearest whole number—for example, $33^1/8$ rounds down to 33, while $32^1/2$ rounds up to 33. If the new rounded number is even (like 30, 32, or 34), then add 4 inches. If it's an odd number (like 31, 33, or 37), add 5 inches. This number is your band size.

To get your cup size, measure all the way around your breasts and chest, at the nipple level (where your breasts are the biggest). Round this number up or down to the nearest whole number. Next subtract your band size from this number. The result is your difference. Write it down. The smaller the difference, the smaller your cup size; the larger the difference, the bigger your cup size.

Cup size goes up with each additional 1-inch difference: an A cup is for a 1-inch difference, a B cup for a 2-inch difference, a C cup for a 3-inch difference, a D cup for a 4-inch difference, a DD cup or E cup for a 5-inch difference, a DDD cup or F cup for a 5-inch difference, a DDDD cup or G cup for a 7-inch difference, and on from there.

Measuring yourself is not so easy, right? Now you can see why it helps for someone else to do this! By the way, it doesn't cost anything to work with a bra fitter—even though you might feel obligated to buy a bra from her after she helps you out. Only buy the bra if it's right for you. And it's only right if you really like the way it looks, fits, and feels.

Strap Size

Nearly all bras come with adjustable straps; they don't have a specific size. The fit of your bra and the length of its straps are supposed to hold your breasts in a position midway between your shoulders and your elbows.

Adjusting bra straps is annoying because the strap adjusters are usually in the back and hard to reach while you're wearing the bra. The bra makers put them in the back because that's really the only place the metal or plastic adjusters will lie flat against your skin and not dig in, the way they would if they were located on your shoulders. But if you're really petite, then the adjusters may end up on top of your shoulders anyway and be uncomfortable, particularly when you carry a heavy book bag or shoulder bag.

For girls with larger breasts, look for a bra with wider straps that don't stretch much. With a wider strap, the weight of your breasts is distributed over a larger area and you'll be more comfortable. The smaller the strap, the more likely it is to dig into your shoulders. Some larger-sized bras have double straps for extra support.

Avoid very thin straps—they give little support and tend to slide down.

girl to girl

Have you ever made your bra straps so short and tight that they dig into your shoulders and the band gets hiked up your back? I've done this so many times, and it wasn't until recently that I realized I was just wearing the wrong bra size. I tightened the straps because the band was too loose around the rib cage. The next time I went bra shopping, I tried on a bra one band size smaller and also went up a cup size. Bingo! I went from a 34C to a 32D. I've been well supported ever since!

Buying a Bra: Finding the Right Fit

The first step to buying a bra is figuring out your correct bra size. The best way to get an accurate measurement of your breasts is to be fitted by a person who knows what she's doing.

Bra fitters can be found in most lingerie stores or in the bra section of a department store. You can usually walk in and meet with a fitter, but just to be sure that one is available to help you, it's best to call in advance and make an appointment.

If you're too embarrassed to have a bra fitter in the changing room with you, don't worry. Measuring girls' chests and checking out how the bras actually fit on you are what a bra fitter does every day, all day long—just think about how many breasts she's seen! But if you want to be super-private, she can measure you with clothes or a bra on, and then pass the bras over the dressing room curtain or door for you to try on. But you won't get the best fit that way.

If you have very small breasts or are getting your first bra, the best measurement is done with nothing on from the waist up. If you have more mature breasts that are large or sit lower, the breast tissue tends to be spread out between your chest and upper belly area. That's why the most accurate measurements are done when your breasts are together with a bra on (non-padded).

If you have a small frame, an adult bra might be too big for you, so look for a youth bra. Bra brands and styles can fit differently. So make sure to try on various bra sizes as you shift from one brand and style to the next.

To make sure a bra fits right, you should keep in mind two important things: how the bra wears and how your body changes affect fit.

First, bras stretch out as you wear them. They can be tightened or loosened using the three rows of hooks in the back. A bra that fits perfectly on the tightest row when you buy it, though, might become too big after even a few weeks of wear because you can't hook it any tighter to take up any slack.

Second, it's best to buy a bra that fits when it's hooked in the middle row, so if you gain or lose weight, the bra will adjust with you. It's also a good choice if your breasts are still growing and you need room to grow.

But if you think you've stopped growing, buy a bra that fits snugly on the first row of hooks (tightest fit), because it's likely to loosen up and fit just right over time.

FYI, bras that fasten in the front often have only one row of hooks and are hard to adjust if the bra stretches out or if your weight goes up or down.

Also, make sure that the middle of the bra, between your breasts, lies flat against your chest. That's where the underwires come together if it's an underwire bra. Sometimes there's just a stiff panel of fabric there.

In the Dressing Room

While in the dressing room, test out the bra to see if it works. Adjust the straps so they stay up and give support. Then jump up and down a few times. Dance around a bit. Stretch and twist. Does the bra stay in place? Do the hooks pop open? Do your breasts pop out? Do the straps fall down? Does the bra dig in anywhere?

Once you find your size, you can go around the sales floor and search for bras yourself, or you can ask the fitter to bring you a few.

Make sure to tell the fitter exactly what you're interested in buying. Are you buying a bra for a specific outfit, like a dress for a special event? Be sure to bring the special dress or top with you to try on over the bra. Are you looking for a push-up bra? Or do you just want an everyday bra? Be as specific as possible so the sales associate can bring you exactly what you're looking for.

Once you've found a bra that you are thinking of buying, you should try on a shirt over it to make sure it gives you the desired look. Even though a bra might look very pretty without a shirt on, you'll be wearing it *under* your clothes. For example, a pretty lace bra can look lumpy under a shirt. You may even want to bring another shirt with you to test out how it looks under different types of clothing. Doing this will help predict whether you'll wear the bra or if it will just sit in your drawer.

Picking the Best Bra Style for You

After you've found the right size, it's time to try out some of the different styles of bra. Through trial (and maybe error) you'll hit on one or more styles that fit your "girls" best. The great thing about shopping for bras nowadays is having lots of choices.

Here are some of the most popular types of bras that you'll find:

- TRAINING BRA. Your first bra might be a training bra. It's called a training bra *not* because it is training your breasts to grow (sorry!) but because it helps you get used to wearing a bra every day. A training bra is usually a snug-fitting half-camisole made out of a thin, comfortable fabric. Even if you don't need major support, these kinds of bras are great for flattening out puffy nipples so they don't show through clothing. Training bras usually come in sizes extra-small through extra-large instead of cup and band sizes like 32A or 38C.

- CAMI BRA. A simple and comfortable bra is the full or half cami (short for *camisole*). It looks like a tight sleeveless undershirt. The half cami with elastic at the bottom is a popular type of training bra. A form-fitting camisole with an attached bra shelf underneath is a popular way to wear a tank top without a bra (whose straps can show or fall down). Girls of any size can wear this style. If you have large breasts, a simple shelf underneath is unlikely to give you enough support, however, several bra companies make a tank top with a full bra underneath to give you that extra support.

> *girl to girl*
>
> My aunt tried to get me to hand a bra to my cousin during a family gathering. "Go over and just give it to her," she said. "Her father won't notice."
>
> "I'll do it my way," I told my aunt.
>
> I would never want to be told in front of my dad to wear a bra.

- UNDERWIRE. An underwire bra has a C-shaped wire sewn into the bottom of each cup that rests in the crease below your breasts. The wire gives the bra more strength and structure, and in turn the bra gives your breasts more solid support. If the bra fits properly, it should be comfortable to wear. If the underwire is too big or too wide, it can dig into your side or armpit. If it's too small, it can push into your breasts. Sometimes, after you've worn and washed a bra a lot, the underwire can stick out of its tunnel and poke you—ouch! Don't wear it again unless you sew it back into its tunnel.

- MOLDED CUP AND THIN-CUP BRAS. Molded bras have cups with a preset shape and size made of several layers of fabric and sometimes foam. When you wear this type of bra, your breasts take on the size and shape of its cups. Girls with very small breasts or narrow breasts often prefer a molded cup because it can enhance their size and round out their shape. This type of bra also helps hide big nipples.

In contrast, thin-cup bras are made with just one or two layers of soft, stretchy fabric. Their flexible cups take on your breasts' unique size and shape. If your breasts are still growing, a thin-cup bra can "grow" (stretch) with you. You can find styles with and without underwires.

- PADDED AND PUSH-UP BRAS. Padded bras have extra foam and fabric inside the cups to make your breasts look bigger. Some bras have padding that's sewn into the cup, and others have removable pads that fit into a pocket within the cup. Push-up bras have extra padding in the bottom of the cups in order to push your breasts up and together to create cleavage. These types of bras usually have a molded cup.

- ATHLETIC OR SPORTS BRAS. Athletic bras are designed to give you maximum support and comfort while you are most active. Sports bras are constructed out of thick but slightly stretchy material to hold your breasts in tight and also allow you to move in comfort.

They have a racer back so you don't have to worry about the straps falling off your shoulders.

Some sports bras that are specially designed for large breasts may have underwires for added support. If you think you need one of these, double-check to see if the wire is securely sewed in. The last thing you want is a sharp wire poking you in the middle of a soccer game.

- STRAPLESS AND CONVERTIBLE BRAS. A strapless bra has cups and a band designed to stay in place and provide enough support without straps so you can wear strapless sundresses and tops. A convertible bra is approximately the same shape as a strapless bra, except it has removable straps. You can convert the strap style to fit your needs— halter style, crisscross-back style, single-strap for a one-sleeved shirt, and many other combinations. It's easy to lose the straps, though, so keep the straps together with the bra in a corner of your drawer.

- RACER-BACK BRAS. Racer-back bras are practical because the straps don't fall off your shoulders. This style bra usually hooks in the front between your breasts (or has no hooks). The straps connect the top of each cup to a panel of fabric in the middle of your back, and that panel is attached to the band. Most sports bras are made with a racer back so you don't have to worry about fiddling with your straps in the middle of a game.

- SPECIAL BRAS. Lots of bras are designed for special occasions. There is a low-back bra for a dress or top with a very low back. A backless bra attaches to your sides with stickers. There are also sticky gel cups that stick to your breasts and just provide a little cover without any real support.

If you're wearing a special outfit (like a prom dress) that won't allow a regular bra, you may need a custom solution. If you just want nipple coverage, you can buy special stickers to put over your nipples. These are called *pasties* or *petals*. If you also need support, you might be able to use a special kind of bra discussed above. Or you could get resourceful and sew one of your bras into the dress. This usually requires cutting the bra to fit the dress, but it's worth it for a very special occasion, particularly if you're going to wear the dress a few times (save your money and just use one of your older bras for this).

If you have a dress that makes you look flat and no bra will fit underneath it but you want some breast shape, you can sew pads into the dress.

- BRA COLOR AND PATTERN. Pink, turquoise, name the color—you can have a lot of fun wearing bras with different colors and prints. Animal-print ones can look wild, and others can look like a costume, full of lace, flowers, and ribbons.

  You don't want your bra to show through or stick out from under your clothes. Bringing attention to your bra is asking for the wrong kind of attention. (Some boys and men will notice your bra immediately and get all kinds of ideas, which is not good or safe for you.)

  The best color of bra to wear depends on what you're wearing over it. If your shirt is a solid dark color, wear whatever bra color you want. If you are wearing a light-colored or thin top, then wear a skin-colored bra that's thick enough to hide your nipples and areolas. Over the years, you'll find that skin-colored bras are the most practical because they can be worn with anything. Black and animal print bras can make you feel grown-up and are fun to wear. Enjoy them as long as they don't show ☺.

Bra Comfort Is Key

Bra comfort is just as important as bra fit. If your bra fits correctly, it should not be painful or uncomfortable to wear. When a bra doesn't fit properly, you can get back and shoulder aches, neck discomfort, and little dents in your shoulders—particularly if you're large-breasted.

Your bra needs to be comfortable both physically and mentally. A bra may be supportive, but if it makes your breasts look way too big for your comfort level, that's no good! Here are a few bra problems you may run into that might make you feel self-conscious or embarrassed:

- Your nipples show through an unlined bra.

- The colorful pattern on your bra is visible through a shirt.

- A lace bra makes your breasts look lumpy.

- The bra cups are too close together and push your breasts up against each other.

- Your breasts look too big or too small.

To do sports, you need a bra that's comfortable, doesn't rub anywhere, and holds you nice and tight when you're running around. Avoid seams inside the cup that might rub against sensitive places, like your nipples.

Bras come in many different fabrics. Soft fabrics that are thick and stiff enough to give you good support will provide the most comfort. If your breasts get bigger before your menstrual period, choose a bra with stretchy enough cups to handle the extra size (or you might need to get a bigger bra just for that time of the month). If you're looking for nipple coverage, choose a bra with a thick-walled cup. There are also things you can insert into your bra to cover big nipples, such as *dimmers* (for your "headlights"). Stores such as Victoria's Secret offer all of these products.

Any Questions?

How do I know if I'm wearing the right size bra?
A bra is too big if the band is too loose, your breasts don't fill in the cups, or the straps are too long even when all of these parts are fully tightened. A bra is too small if the band is too tight and digs into your rib cage, your breasts or nipples are popping out of the cups, or the straps are too short even when they are fully lengthened. The right size bra will feel so comfortable that you don't even think about it, but it will provide the support you need for your everyday activities.

If my breasts are lopsided, what size bra do I buy?

All bras are made with two identical-sized cups. So if you're a size A on one side and a C on the other side, you should buy a bra to fit the biggest breast and then find a solution to fill in the cup that's too big (where your smaller breast is).

Using a pad on the smaller side is an easy adjustment. Pads come in all different shapes and sizes and have all sorts of names: *pad, lift, curve, cutlet,* or *cookie.* You can buy them at most bra and department stores. One popular solution is to buy a padded bra with removable pads and take out the pad on the bigger side. If needed, you can add this extra pad to the smaller side to even you out further. Make sure to secure the pads into your bra so they don't fall out.

The one thing you *don't* want to do is put cotton balls or tissues in your bra to fill it out. They can make your breasts look bumpy, or even worse, they can fall out—an embarrassing moment to avoid!

Can I wear a bathing suit top instead of a bra?

It's okay to wear a bathing suit top instead of a bra on occasion. Bathing suit tops are designed to fit against your body and dry off quickly after getting wet. But they're not meant to give much support; they don't look as good under clothes, and they don't increase airflow, so you sweat more in them.

How should I wash my bras?

All day long, sweat and anything you put on your skin (deodorant, perfume, lotion) gets on your bra. That's why it's best to wash your bra after each use.

Washing your bras requires extra care because they are delicate and made of many pieces. To make them last and stay strong and supportive, it's best to wash a bra by hand in cool or warm water—but it may be too hard to find time to do this. The next best thing is to wash your bras in the washing machine on the delicate or hand-wash setting. First fasten the bra hooks and put them into a mesh lingerie-washing bag. This keeps them from snagging, tangling, twisting, tearing, and getting bent out of shape. Use a mild lingerie soap (such as Forever New) and avoid regular detergents (even Woolite).

After washing, hang the bras to dry over a hanger, hook, or door-knob. Don't put them in the dryer! The heat and tumble of a dryer are too rough on a bra's elastic, embroidery, and lace.

How many bras do I need?

You need at least three bras: one to wear, one in the laundry, and one in your dresser ready for tomorrow. How many more bras you need depends on how fast your breasts are growing, how often you do your laundry, and how many bras you use each day (if you do sports, you might wear more than one bra each day). If your breasts are growing really fast, you might need to go bra shopping every few months. Buy bras that can stretch to accommodate your breasts as they grow, like a thin-cup bra with several hook positions.

If you love to wear strapless tops or dresses, you'll need a strapless bra along with your everyday bras. If you feel that you need many bras to work with all of your different outfits, try a convertible bra.

Do I need to get remeasured once my breasts have finished growing?

Yes! Get remeasured every six to twelve months. Your body is constantly changing, and you want to have a bra that fits and supports your breasts as you develop.

Even if your main breast growth has finished, your breasts may continue to change. They can get wider and fuller over time, increasing your cup size. A weight loss or gain of five pounds or more can affect bra size. Many of us gain and lose this much weight at different times of the month, so you might want to have a bigger bra around for those bigger days. But if your weight changes are larger and last longer, it might be time to get remeasured.

Why do my bra straps keep falling down?

If you have sloping shoulders or if the bra straps are set wide apart, they can slip off your shoulders even at the perfect length. Straps are more likely to stay up when they are close together in the back, as with racer-back and halter-style bras. Some bras have several different places to attach the strap, or you can cut, move, and sew them so that they're closer together in the back. If you get really frustrated with your straps, get a strapless bra, or get a convertible bra and crisscross the straps in the back.

Where can I find a pretty and comfortable bra for very large breasts? (One that doesn't look like my grandmother's!)

It used to be hard to find attractive, supportive, and comfortable bras for girls with big breasts. But the good news is that more and more companies are making them, including Wacoal, Elila, Goddess, Lunaire, Naturana, Fantasie, Freya, and Chantelle. For more reasonably priced plus sizes, check out Just My Size bras.

If you're big-breasted, you require extra support to be comfortable. A poorly fitting bra can lead to back, shoulder, and neck strain—and sometimes headaches. The weight of your breasts has to be properly distributed between the band, cups, and straps, and each of these parts must be made of relatively stiff fabric in order to provide the best support. (Stretchy fabrics let you bounce all around.) Underwire bras provide more structure and support, but look for ones with foam-wrapped wires so they are comfortable.

If there is no specialty bra store around you (such as the Town Shop in New York City), you can usually find bras in your size at Internet sites such as Figleaves.com, Brasmyth.com, and Justmysize.com (or jms.com).

What bras can make me look smaller?

You may choose a "minimizer" bra if you have very big breasts and you want them to look smaller. But simply wearing a very good, supportive bra can make your breasts look a bit smaller, and you'll look a lot slimmer with a bra that lifts your breasts up, showing off your waist.

Bras for You

Should I wear a bra at night?

Wearing a bra at night is unnecessary and can be uncomfortable. If you've been wearing a bra all day, it's best to give your breasts some freedom at night. If you fall asleep with your bra on, at least unhook it if you don't have the energy to slip it off.

Some girls like to wear a bra at night to keep their breasts together while sleeping. Sleeping bras or night bras are different from daytime bras. They are usually made of one layer of soft fabric, hook in the front, and provide very little support.

Does wearing a bra or sleeping with a bra cause breast cancer or stop your breasts from growing?

Wearing a bra or sleeping with a bra on does *not* stop the growth of your breasts and does *not* increase the risk of breast cancer. The healthiest way to wear a bra is to make sure it's comfortable and fits properly. For full blood flow, circulation of fluids, and the health of your breast tissue, it's important to have time off from the pressure of wearing a bra at night. So it's best to go braless at night. If you feel compelled to wear something to hold you together, try a simple form-fitting T-shirt or camisole instead (so there's no elastic digging in anywhere). And if you can't give up wearing a bra at night, be sure to get a soft nighttime bra, rather than a more structured and tight daytime bra.

What if your mom wants you to buy a different bra than the one you want?

Girls and their moms often disagree about what kind of bra to buy. But if you follow the tips in this section, then you'll be able to figure out what's best for you: a bra that fits, gives you support, and is comfortable. Of course, a nice-looking bra is also important to many girls. When it comes to the price and how much bra is showing, however, you and your mom have to work it out and find a compromise.

You can share your stories at TakingCareOfYourGirls.com.

I'm getting more comfortable with having breasts. I would never show cleavage, but every now and then—no, a lot—I will wear a shirt that you can see that I have them.

Maggie, 14

9

Show Off, Cover Up, or Glide By?

Dress to Express and Move with Confidence

My friend and I were shopping for dresses with her mom, and I was trying on a dress that was pretty low-cut, and my friend's mom said that because I was so much more endowed than my friend I couldn't wear that dress.

Alex, 18

I feel very embarrassed whenever I wear a bikini or tank top because there's always that one person who will tell me that either I need a boob job or need to cover up my chest before I catch a cold.

Isabelle, 14

In class we were talking about breasts and my teacher said we should not wear tight or low-cut tops because it's gonna get all the boys' juices pumping.

Cameron, 12

Each piece of clothing is different for me: some make my breasts look smaller, while other types of shirts make them look bigger. It all really depends.

Olivia, 15

taking care of your "girls"

We have a dress code in school. Shirt necklines must be at or higher than your collarbone. When your arms are raised, your belly can't show. All shorts must be to the knees or longer. Most girls stick to the rules, but of course a few wear revealing stuff to school anyway. They avoid teachers so they don't get caught. Every once in a while, you'll see one of the girls wearing her gym clothes: she got caught!

Suzanna, 12

Although the sweatshirt is the fastest cover-up solution, I still love nice clothes. The cool girls in the class have tons of nice clothes, and I don't want them to think that they are the only ones who get to wear nice things. So whenever I get the courage, I will wear something nice that's more revealing. If I do, then I'll also wear a headband or a belt—something to distract from the breast area.

Lena, 14

My boyfriend's mom told me a story once about her boob popping out of her dress during a formal event. At the prom, she leaned over because she dropped her fork, and the sleeve slid down, which led to her boob popping out (which gave the nice stranger sitting next to her a great view). She told me that when buying a dress, I should always make sure that whichever way I turn, I don't fall out. As if she needed to tell me *that* after her story!

McKenzie, 18

I'm very, very small, so a padded bra and a V-neck (but not too low) shirt looks the best on me. I only buy dark colors: black, brown, navy, dark red, or dark pink—but I would never, ever wear light colors like white or yellow (they show too much).

Lori, 17

My mother and I both have large breasts. She has a very nice figure but always hid it with boxy clothes—and she never bought me anything fitted either. Every sweater hung from my shoulders and nothing showed off my waist. When you're curvy like that, if you have something that doesn't fit around your waist, you just look like a box. It was only after I kind of grew up a bit that I actually started choosing clothes that show my figure.

Rochelle, 19

When you're really tall you feel that you stick out, and you're just starting all this change, so I didn't want people to notice. That's why I started hunching over a little more. It was the only way, I thought, to hide it, even though it just made me feel more uncomfortable. But when I started middle school, there were some older kids around me. I started standing up a little more and eventually I stood up straight.

Ariane, 15

Don't try to blend in—blend out!

Lasayo, 15

First Things First

Can you believe how much time it can sometimes take to get dressed? Whether it's for school each day or a more special occasion, everyone wants to look good and be comfortable. Figuring out the best way to present yourself and your new and growing "girls" to the world can involve many decisions. No wonder you might find yourself running late more often.

Sometimes dealing with your new breasts can be a problem—that snug T-shirt you've had since fourth grade isn't looking so great anymore. But your brother's huge sweatshirt isn't a very good choice either. During puberty and beyond, every time you look in the mirror, your breasts might seem too big, too small, too flat, too pointy—the sky's the limit for negative feelings.

It doesn't help that many of the girls and young women on TV and in magazines are much thinner than the average person. No wonder after a few hours of TV or flipping through a fashion magazine we feel bad about our own bodies. Girls shouldn't have to limit their body expectations to everything that's broadcast through the media. All those pictures are designed to be super-beautiful, not realistic. A 10-year-old girl shouldn't think her breasts are too small because of a picture of a model in a magazine that has been airbrushed, Photoshopped, and otherwise doctored. And a 14-year-old shouldn't think her butt is too big because of a celebrity makeover show.

Starting right now, you need to throw away your bad feelings about your body. This chapter will show you and your "girls" how to look your best for your unique size and shape. As Finola Hughes, host of the Style Network show *How Do I Look,* says, "The biggest mistake girls make is to wear clothing that's too big."

The best approach is to dress the body that you have today and celebrate it. We'll help you carry yourself with style and find things that look good, fit your personal taste, are fun to wear, build your self-esteem, and command respect from others.

Here's the Scoop

Girls in our survey suggested that if your breasts are really small, show them off by wearing tight, low-cut clothes and a padded or push-up bra. If your breasts are really big, hide them in loose, baggy, dark clothing. But you probably have a lot more choices besides these two extremes of showing them off or hiding them away.

Whether you are big-breasted or have smaller proportions, here are a few simple guidelines to help you look your best—for school, for special occasions, for whenever!

Keep It Vertical

The bigger breasts get, the more the eye goes from side to side rather than up and down. That's why girls with very large breasts look wider and shorter than they really are. The solution: emphasize the vertical lines of your clothing to minimize attention to the breast area and make yourself look tall and slender. Clothing that makes the eye go up and down, along your center (imagine a line between your eyes, along your nose, and through your belly button) is most flattering for girls who have large breasts and/or short waists. Choose clothes with:

- Vertical stripes

- Vertical seams—such as princess seams, which start at your armpits, arch around the breast area, and swoop vertically down to the level of your hips

- Buttons down the front

- A zipper in front

- V-shaped necklines

- The same dark color from top to bottom, using light or bright colors in the middle (like a bright tank top under a dark cardigan)

- Small prints (avoid big prints, which make you look wide)

- Fitted tops (no big sweatshirts)

- Boot-cut or flared-leg jeans (they help pull the eye all the way down)

For girls who have a pear shape—that is, a body that is narrow on top and wider on the bottom—a different set of rules apply. Choose clothes with:

- Horizontal striped tops (to even out your top with your bottom)

- Fitted waists (to give your upper body a curvier shape)

- Shoulder pads (to make narrow or sloping shoulders look wider, which shows off your waist)

- Bold patterns (to make your narrow parts appear a little wider)

No matter what your shape is, make sure your clothes continue to fit as your breasts grow. You will have to give up some old favorites when they become too small.

Under It All

Good undergarments are also absolutely essential to looking good in clothes. They shape and make you look more slender. A good bra lifts the "girls"—especially if you have large ones. This makes your torso look longer and curvier (read more about your bra options in Chapter 8). You will be amazed, too, by how much a good bra can help smooth out any bumps or rolls you may have on your torso (which can make you look wider and shorter than you really are).

Steering People's Attention?

You can direct people's attention to where you want it to go with the clothing you choose. Details automatically draw people's attention, near or far from the breast area: buttons, ruffles, embroidery, pockets, or bright contrasting trim, for example. You can purchase tops with details in the right spots or place details on tops you already have. You can also get other pieces of clothing or accessories to direct people's attention to other areas, such as big earrings or a big belt, bold big sunglasses, a funky hairband or a fun necklace (pick one that's closer to your neck than to your cleavage), jeans with embroidery, or fancy boots.

There are other details that can take the focus off your breasts, whatever size they are. Try textured or crinkled fabric, bright colors or patterned fabrics with stripes, or designs like floral, paisley, plaid, or animal prints (leopard, zebra, snake). The eye concentrates on the pattern itself, not what the fabric is covering.

Fabrics can be sewn in a way that distracts people's attention from your breasts, such as ruching (small gathers of fabric), pleating (folds of fabric), and ruffles. For instance, if you wear a scoopneck top with a ruffle around the neckline, the eye will be drawn to the detail and your collarbone area.

The opposite is also important to keep in mind. There are many styles that bring attention straight to your breasts. Low necklines that fall into your cleavage or T-shirts with messages written on the front bring the eye straight to the breast area. When you wear a colored bra under a see-through top, your bra shows and will quickly get people's attention.

For both big- and small-breasted girls, layering works great. Layers can deemphasize the breasts. Try a button-down shirt over a tank top or a jean jacket over a T-shirt. A vest looks good over a top with a detail in the middle like a ruffle or a scarf. If you choose to layer, select layers made of thin, well-fitting fabrics or your shape will get lost in the layers. Thick layers also make you look big—and too warm. Bulky and sweaty? No thanks!

For bigger-busted girls, draping fabrics in the right places can work. Try a top or dress that drapes over the breasts but comes in tighter at your waist with elastic or a tie. Be careful, though—it's easy for your shape to get lost in the extra fabric.

girl to girl

I have a friend who is the queen of layering. She has big boobs, but you'd never know it by the way she dresses, and she likes it that way. She usually wears a couple of layered tank tops with a colorful zip-up sweatshirt over it. All her layers are fitted, including the sweatshirt, so she still looks great. The look takes attention off her breasts and really shows off her legs.

Flirty, Sexy Looks

If you're shooting for a sexy look, more is not necessarily better. If you push up your breasts to create super-cleavage in a really low-cut shirt, everyone will be staring at you, and that probably isn't the kind of attention you want.

There are other ways to create a flirty and tasteful look. Try different fabrics, such as satin, silk, and knits that fit your curves in just the right way.

Showing off other parts of your body can be really attractive too. Complement your collarbones with an interesting neckline and a simple necklace. Find a top that is cut low in the back for a surprising and flirty look. If you love your legs, wear a pair of boots with fitted jeans to show them off.

> ### girl to girl
>
> Speaking of breasts and accessories, I've discovered some cool ways to accessorize my breasts. I'm a big-time scarf wearer and I've found that they complement my breasts very well. Sometimes I wear a long silk scarf around my neck. It brings attention to my face, elongates my figure, and frames my breasts nicely.

Think of your breasts as accessories. You wouldn't wear all of your rings and handbags at once; you wear them in moderation. The same thing goes with wearing your breasts: wear them to complement the rest of your look.

Check Your Packaging Before Going out the Door

You're in control of the kind of attention you want to attract to yourself. So before you head out the door in the morning, take a good look at yourself and make sure your clothing choices say what you want them to say. Choose your clothes carefully, not only so that others respect you but also so that you are comfortable, pleased with how you look, and proud of yourself.

Like it or not, first impressions say a lot. Before you get to know someone, you only have the most obvious traits available to make a first judgment. People often make fast judgments based on the clothes you're wearing and how you carry yourself. There are all kinds of attraction, but whether you want to attract attention from a parent, teacher, sibling, or crush, you want to put your best foot forward.

Show Off, Cover Up, or Glide By?

If you wear clothes that show self-respect and you wear them with confidence, you are more likely to receive the same respect from others. Establishing a good first impression from the get-go in any situation is to your advantage.

Sometimes a certain outfit can be perceived differently by you and by others. If you're wearing a top that you love because it's super-comfortable, but it's low-cut and shows off your cleavage, some people might assume that your intentions are sexual, even if they're not.

Some factors of attraction are completely out of your control. Another aspect of how people respond to you is their own intentions—completely colored by what they think, want, and imagine. You have very little control over these things. But if you give them the opportunity to imagine what they want and are looking for, then they will seize the opportunity.

Given the weirdo factor out there, if you do ever wear stuff that's revealing, be sure to have a cardigan or cover-up with you to throw on if you find some creep staring at you.

With all that said, don't base what you wear on what other people will think of you. Put out the image that you want to put out, and above all, maintain your individuality. We want you to make the impression you want to make, attract the right attention, and be aware of the range of reactions you can receive.

Stand Up for Your "Girls"

How you stand and move can really affect how you and your "girls" look, and the impression you give. It's pretty common for girls to hunch their

> ## girl to girl
>
> I hate superficial judgments more than anything else! But the truth is that before you *really* get to know someone, much of your perception is shaped by clues given off from clothing and the way someone carries herself—we're all guilty of it. I don't alter what I like to wear to fit what other people think. I am just myself. Sometimes I get respect from others, and sometimes I don't. But at the end of the day I can come home and say I stayed true to who I am and who I want to be, and that's something to feel good about.

shoulders and not stand up straight. This is particularly true for girls who are tall or who have either very big or very small breasts. The problem is that hunching over hurts your back, looks bad, and makes you appear insecure. It becomes a bad habit that's hard to break. Over the years, it can cause back discomfort, neck pain, headaches, even trouble breathing (it's hard to take deep breaths when your chest is curled over).

The good news is that you are young enough to do something about it before it becomes a problem. First, actively resist the temptation to hunch over. Train your body to stand, sit, and move around with good posture. Focus mainly on these two things: Stand or sit *straight,* with your shoulders back directly over your hips and your head in line with your spine—not leaning over in front (stand against a wall to see what straight really feels like). Likewise, stand or sit *tall.* Push your feet down against the floor and also stretch your head up toward the ceiling. Imagine a string pulling the top of your head up like a puppet on a string. But don't exaggerate these movements, or else you'll look like a walking wooden board!

Yoga, ballet, and other dance classes are great ways to improve your posture and the way you carry yourself. Get a group of friends together and take one of these classes.

> ## girl to girl
>
> A few summers ago, I made a conscious effort to have good posture. I wrote on my hand "SUS," which stood for "stand up straight," and whenever I caught myself slouching, I straightened up. I was so persistent with myself that I finally stopped slouching altogether. Now, I stand up straight and tall and all that work definitely paid off. Having good posture makes me feel more strong and confident. Sometimes people even comment on how good my posture is.

Any Questions?

People tell me that I have big boobs. I don't think they're big. But it kind of makes me self-conscious. Any suggestions?

It's great that you feel comfortable with your breast size. Ignore these big-mouthed friends who are talking about big boobs. Go right ahead and enjoy fitted, flattering clothes that make you look both terrific and respectable. Get a good bra, try some layers and have fun with accessories. Do *not* hide. And when you walk around, stand up straight, glide by these people, and be confident in yourself and your breasts.

Can a good bra help with my posture?

If you talk to any bra specialist, they'll tell you that good posture definitely depends on the right-fitting bra. Breasts can be very heavy and really need to be supported—a size D breast weighs about two and a half pounds, so you're talking about five pounds that a bra is going to pull down against your shoulders and your neck muscles. As strong as they are, bras can get stressed from supporting all of the weight. Dan Koch, owner of a specialty bra store called the Town Shop in New York City, says, "With the wrong size bra on, you may be hunched over, but when you get fitted for the right size you look totally different. Part of it is that your breasts are sitting where they're supposed to sit. It's amazing. I tell my clients, 'Look at you.' And they go, 'I know, I know.' Their whole presentation of their body is different after they get the right size."

Is there a special brace that can help me stand up straight?

Your doctor or physical therapist may recommend wearing a special posture brace to keep your shoulders back and your back straight (you wear it under your clothes). It can teach your body better positioning and help it remember the new healthier posture. Eventually the training and effort pay off with long-term improvement in your posture. Then later you can use the brace only occasionally, as a physical backup. You can buy a brace from a specialty drugstore or online, but before you wear it, make sure it fits properly and that it's not too tight or restrictive. Don't wear one without first checking with your doctor.

There's a lot of pressure at school to look sexy. I want to fit in and have fun too.

All around the world, breasts are a sex symbol and a source of attraction and attention (wanted and unwanted).

But looking sexy mostly comes from how attractive you feel on the inside and how you express it on the outside. Showing a lot of cleavage doesn't automatically give you a sexy look. In fact, if too much of your "girls" are hanging out, it can turn off or bring on the wrong kind of response from others. More important than being and feeling sexy is simply being and feeling attractive.

The key to looking and feeling attractive is to feel good about yourself and feel confident in how you look. Showing a lot of cleavage does not have to be part of the equation. Wearing fun clothes that fit your body properly and that work with your own personal style is essential. Attraction is multifaceted and does not depend on the appearance of your breasts or any other single body part. Confidence in your whole self, body and mind, is of utmost importance.

Sometimes—okay, often—I compare myself to other girls.
How can I stop?

We've all compared ourselves with someone else at some point in our lives. It's just human nature. Unfortunately, we tend to be overly critical of ourselves. As a friend says, we each have an "itty bitty critty committee" that always criticizes the way we look and has nothing nice to say. It's a little voice that says negative stuff like, "Oh, your breasts are too saggy," "Ugh, you look like a boy," "You look fat all over," or "Your boobs are gi-normous." You have to toss that committee and hire your own cheerleading squad.

You'll always be able to find someone else who you think looks better than you or who has something that you don't have. Too much jealousy or envy can distract you from your own great qualities and make you feel bad about yourself. Forgive yourself for the jealousy—we all deal with it—and move on. It's *your* life, after all, that counts to you and to everyone who loves you.

You can share your stories at TakingCareOfYourGirls.com.

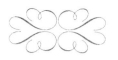

Are there any ways I could make my breasts bigger? I want my prom dress and dressy shirts to show a little cleavage. I'm nervous about asking anyone else, because I'm very self-conscious about my chest. Don't get me wrong, I'm happy with my body, and I know that small isn't always bad, but I would like to enhance myself.

Lauren, 17

10

When You Want Your Breast Size to Be Different:

From Padded Bras to Surgery

One of my best friends has a very small frame but size 36DD breasts. Although she has gotten used to them, the weight of her breasts often hurts her back and she wears both an underwire bra and a sports bra every single day.

Alexandra, 17

When my breasts stopped growing at age 17, I was 5'3" and broad-shouldered, with a 40E bra size. Basically, I was ready to have surgery because I couldn't stand it anymore. It was painful to run (besides the fact that everyone would stare at me). I was starting to have physical problems in the rest of my body in addition to the emotional effects. Like, I was getting dents in my shoulders from my bra straps, my back hurt, and I had scoliosis (curvature of the spine). And that's actually how we got it paid for by our health insurance.

Mara, 19

When my aunt was my age she thought her breasts were way too big so she wore a bra one size too small so they would look smaller.

Chrissy, 19

My breasts are huge and way too big compared to the rest of my body. One day I'm going to turn and knock someone out with them.

Meredith, 18

Well, one of my good friends has really big breasts and she hates them enough to want a reduction. She always tells me she wishes she had the same size boobs as me.

Anya, 15

I wish I had one size bigger boobs so I would be more confident about my body. When I was younger I used to have to get a small bottom and medium top for a bathing suit. Now I have to get a medium bottom and small top. It stinks.

Sara, 14

How do you make breasts bigger naturally (not too big) and right for you in a healthy way (without cosmetic surgery)? How do you know what the right breast size is for you?

Joy, 12

I got a boob job as a sweet-16 present from my parents. They said I was perfect the way I was, but I still got the present. Where I'm from in Texas, it's a thing. Two of my friends had it done first. But I was the one who was real small. If I could tell girls thinking about it one thing, yes, you might look hot after, but surgery hurts. Just because it's not for a serious medical reason doesn't mean the whole hospital thing isn't really serious. The nurses and doctors really put you through a big production.

Britt, 19

what two moms had to say

One of my daughter's breasts never fully developed. It is 80 percent smaller than the fully developed side. It affects her life daily and prevents her from joining in some every-day things. No one at school knows. She avoids bathing suits, sleeveless shirts, and most dresses and gowns. It is very difficult for her. We have been to many doctors. She has learned tremendously from the experience. I have found that my only success in helping her is listening. She feels isolated because I could never understand what she has gone through.

Nancy

My daughter is concerned that hers are too small and two different sizes. I try to re-assure her that this is a very common concern among young girls. I try to always keep the lines of communication open!

Leslie

I had complained to my mother and to my doctor about being completely flat-chested. They knew also that my breasts never grew. But never did they ever tell me I could do something about it. There was nothing in the library—I was so frustrated. Eventually I had surgery. After one week, I never ever, ever, ever, ever regretted it. When my new breasts settled down, it was the first time I had breasts. I was happier than happy.

Lucy, 21

I had breast reduction surgery when I was 19 (I had J-cup jugs and then went down to a C cup). I don't even want to tell you. Then I went and lost a bunch of weight in college when I got onto the varsity soccer team. Guess what? My boobs went down to a small B cup. Now I'm wishing I could go back in time and change things a little.

Katherine, 23

First Things First

All girls have pretty strong feelings about the size and shape of their breasts. The uncertainty of not knowing how big, full, or even their breasts will become makes many girls anxious.

Several thousand girls told us how they feel about their breast size.

- About 75 percent of girls are satisfied with their breast size.

- Another 20 percent of girls feel that their breasts are too small.

- Around 5 percent say that they are too large.

- About 25 percent are concerned about being lopsided.

- Some girls are concerned about having droopy or narrow breasts.

Most girls (about 70 percent) say that their "best breast size" standard comes from their own thinking—but 35–40 percent of girls say that their standard is influenced by images of celebrities, other girls, magazines, movies, and TV.

girl to girl

The way I feel about the size of my breasts depends on the clothes I'm wearing (or want to wear) and my mood. There are some clothes I think would look better if my breasts were smaller and others I think would look better if my breasts were bigger. I have different bras that make my breasts look bigger or smaller, so I pair the right bra with how I want my breasts to look.

Most girls—regardless of how they feel about their breast size—want to know how they can make their breasts *look* smaller or larger without surgery. Less than half of the girls who said their breasts were too big or too small would consider surgery to change their size.

In this chapter we'll tell you about how your breast size and shape can change on its own, and how you can alter your size and shape without (or with) surgery.

Here's the Scoop

It's important to know that your breast size and shape are likely to change through your life. This is natural and normal. As we describe in Chapter 2, you can expect that your breast size and shape will be affected by weight gain and loss, hormone-based medications (such as birth control pills and hormone replacement therapy after menopause), pregnancies, breast-feeding, and changes of weight distribution as you grow older. Some of these changes are temporary, while others are permanent.

Your breasts might stay the same size while the rest of your body changes. For example, maybe you thought your breasts were way too big, but now that you have grown four inches taller and your curves are much fuller, your breasts fit your body quite nicely. Or the opposite can happen—your breasts have gotten bigger but you've stopped growing taller. Perhaps you feel your breasts are too big and way out of proportion to the rest of your body. Or you think they are too small and out of proportion. Some breasts even out and some stay lopsided. There is no correct proportion or perfect breast size. All combinations can work just fine.

How You Feel About Your Breast Size

How you perceive your breast size is complicated. Every girl and woman can find things that she likes and doesn't like about her body, including her breasts. And all of these feeling can change from day to day, depending on what someone says, if your weight is up or down, how things are going in and out of school, whom you look up to, and how you fit into your circle of friends. Styles can also change, and that can affect how you see yourself. One minute, celebrities with large breasts are in; the next minute, models with tiny breasts are admired more. Or a new style comes out that highlights your breast size, which you had previously wanted to change.

girl to girl

Taking care of our minds is just as important as taking care of our bodies. We have doctors for feet, eyes, teeth, and breasts, so think of a therapist as a doctor for your mind. Even though it might seem weird to go to talk to someone about something so personal, a therapist can really help to work out the feelings you have about your body.

The experiences of other women in your family can have a heavy influence on you. Since one of the big factors that determines breast size is genetics, it's likely that other women in your family have faced similar challenges. If you don't like your breasts or feel self-conscious about them, talk to a female family member who has breasts similar to yours. Chances are she'll have some good stories and advice to share, even if the choices you make are different from hers.

Despite all of the changes in your life, you do have the ability to learn to accept and appreciate your breast size as is, without making them bigger or smaller.

Just keep in mind, there is only one you. Your life is your greatest gift, and that includes your body with all of its wonderful elements. There is no perfect breast, body size, or proportion. Focus on the big picture: who you are and what matters most. All of us hear the same thing: try to love and accept yourself. And we each have to work hard to do it. Sometimes it's easier than others. One of the main reasons for writing this book is to encourage you and girls like you to be the best you can be, and to accept and honor yourself along the way.

If you feel like you're hung up on this issue, you may want to see a therapist or school counselor to talk through your feelings about your body. Maybe someone said something mean to you about your breast size, for example, and you can't stop thinking about it. You can work through and resolve any body concerns without doing anything to change your breast size. Work through these difficult issues you might be feeling with someone you trust.

Bust Enhancers: Products and Foods

You might have heard or read about all kinds of things that claim to make breasts bigger, fuller, and firmer—creams, special exercises, suction cup machines, various foods, and pills and supplements. These things don't work! There are no pills or potions proven to safely and effectively enlarge your breasts.

Watch out for solutions that people swear by. Foods that make you gain weight can also make your breasts bigger, but there are no foods that cause weight gain only in the breast area. When I was 12 years old, my slightly older sister and I read a magazine article that promised bigger breasts after a tablespoon a day of olive oil. We followed the "prescription" strictly. Two months later, we'd gained a few pounds and went up a dress size, but our breasts barely got bigger. Bummer!

Likewise, products that claim to minimize big breasts and boost sagging breasts don't work. Some of the pills that claim to "get rid of extra water weight" are unsafe. A really good bra and flattering clothing remain the best solutions.

New products are being promoted all the time, especially on the Internet. But beware of the gimmicks. Advertisements can be full of promises, customers' miracle stories, and false 100 percent money-back guarantees. These products are designed to appeal to women and girls who are self-conscious or insecure about their bodies. Don't be fooled by the ads, as tempting as they make their product out to be—these solutions don't work, and they could even be harmful. Save your money for something worthwhile, like a great pair of shoes.

Special lingerie such as padded bras, push-up bras, or falsies might

girl to girl

I knew a girl who claimed that oatmeal made her breasts bigger! She said that she had been eating a lot of oatmeal recently and she noticed her breasts had gotten bigger. She was a late bloomer, so I think she was just going through her regular breast development, but she was so excited that I didn't have the heart to tell her she was probably wrong about the oatmeal.

make your breasts *look* bigger, though none of these will make your breasts permanently bigger. But these are the easiest and healthiest ways to have fun trying on different breast sizes.

Surgery to Make Breasts Bigger

With all of the plastic surgery shows on TV, you may have wondered what it would be like to have breast surgery. It's very normal and natural to wonder about these kinds of things. By this point in our book, you've gotten to know us pretty well. We enjoy talking to you about all kinds of things openly, but we also have a point of view on many topics. And we do *not* support breast surgery in most situations. It's much easier, safer, and healthier to change your breast size up or down with

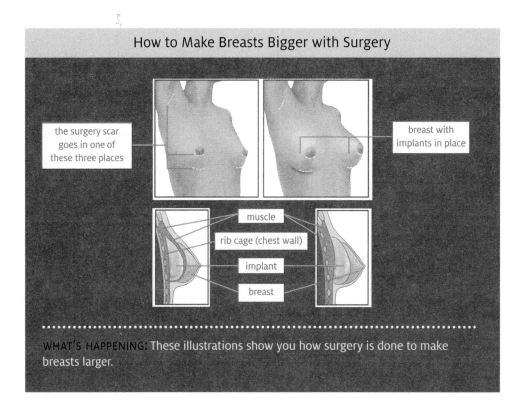

How to Make Breasts Bigger with Surgery

the surgery scar goes in one of these three places

breast with implants in place

muscle

rib cage (chest wall)

implant

breast

WHAT'S HAPPENING: These illustrations show you how surgery is done to make breasts larger.

bras and clothing. But for those of you who are very interested in surgery, you deserve to get solid and accurate information. That's what this section is for.

Most cosmetic breast surgeries are done to make them bigger. This is done by placing an implant behind your breast tissue, usually under your chest muscle, through a small incision. The incision can be made under your breast, around your nipple, in your underarm, or through your navel.

There are two main types of implants: silicone and saline. Both are made with a soft, thick, round plastic bag. A silicone implant is gel-filled, and a saline implant is fluid-filled. There are also some newer implants made with a bag inside the outer bag and filled with other kinds of liquids, such as soybean oil.

During a breast augmentation (implant) surgery, you're put to sleep for a short period of time. A small incision is placed in one of the locations shown in the illustration. The implant goes through the incision and into position behind the breast and chest muscle. After surgery, you can feel pain, tightness, and pressure because your skin, muscle, and breast tissue are stretched out over the implant underneath. Eventually, things ease up, and the discomfort usually goes away. The risk of other complications is low and is discussed later in this section.

> ### girl to girl
>
> Some breast augmentations come out great. You can barely tell that the person has had it done. That should probably be the end goal. The ones that aren't so great are when you are 100 percent sure the person has had a boob job. I go to this dance class and the instructor is very petite but she has gi-normous boobs that don't really move when she dances. It's a little freaky and sad to me, 'cause I like to see women I respect just kind of relying on their natural beauty.

Surgery to Make Breasts Smaller

Girls with very large breasts who are dealing with back and shoulder pain, difficulty running, and self-image issues may seriously consider surgery to make their breasts smaller and more manageable. By presenting this information to you, we are not promoting this or any other

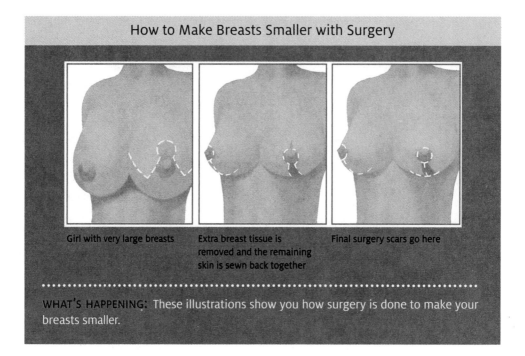

How to Make Breasts Smaller with Surgery

Girl with very large breasts

Extra breast tissue is removed and the remaining skin is sewn back together

Final surgery scars go here

WHAT'S HAPPENING: These illustrations show you how surgery is done to make your breasts smaller.

kind of breast surgery. But we do know that you and your family deserve the best information as you explore your options.

Surgery to reduce breast size takes several steps. It is done under general anesthesia, while you're asleep.

Here are the steps involved: Extra breast tissue and skin are removed from the bottom half of the breasts, the remaining breast tissue is brought to a higher position, the nipple position is moved up, and the skin is sewn back together.

Surgery to Make Breasts More Even

Girls whose breasts remain very lopsided after their breasts have stopped growing may consider surgery to become more even. This is usually done by making the smaller breast bigger, using an implant as described above. Sometimes, if their larger breast is very big, the surgeon may suggest reducing this breast to match the smaller one.

Lift Tips for Droopy Breasts

Girls who have droopy breasts can usually solve their everyday concerns with a very good bra. Upper-body exercises that build up the muscles behind the breast (pectoral muscles) can give you a little lift. But some girls with breasts that sag a great deal may choose to talk to their doctor about getting a breast lift. This procedure is called *mammopexy*. Just as in breast reduction surgery, extra skin is removed from the bottom of the breast, and the nipples/areolas are moved up to a higher position. Similar incisions are used. Breast tissue may or may not be removed, depending on the breast size that you're seeking.

Surgery to Reshape Narrow Breasts

Girls with a very significant form of tubular breasts—when the breasts are very narrow (banana or tube-shaped), set far apart and droopy, and with a puffy areola (described in Chapter 2)—may choose to have surgery. A combination of breast enlargement, reduction, and lift are all required with this type of procedure. The base of the breast is enlarged by opening up the skin and placing an implant, the extra length and droop of the breast is reduced, and the position of the nipples and areolas is raised.

Making the Decision to Change Your Breast Size and Shape with Surgery

This type of surgery is never an emergency, but it is a serious decision that requires careful thought over time. Do some research on your own about options. If this is something that you are seriously considering, it's important to make this decision together with your parents, your regular doctor, and a plastic surgeon who specializes in breast surgery.

You really have to be 100 percent sure you want to do this, as surgery is permanent. Breast-reducing and breast-lifting surgeries *cannot* be undone. Implants can be removed, but there can be leftover side effects such as surgery scars and discomfort.

While we know that you might be thinking about these types of procedures during puberty (and some girls choose to have surgery for their sweet 16), we believe that you really should be at least 18, and preferably quite a bit older, before making the decision to have surgery. As you grow up, your thoughts, tastes, and feelings can change. Your natural breast size and shape can also change into your 20s.

Breast size surgery is not a healthy way to "fix" low self-esteem. How you feel about your breast size can change drastically. You might hate being small-breasted today but love it in only a few years. Having huge breasts might feel like a terrible burden now, but you might change your mind after getting the right bras and figure-friendly clothes. Body "flaws" can be temporary and can be addressed by diet and exercise, as well as smart clothing choices.

Knowing the Risks

Any kind of surgery involves risks. During the surgery, there are always risks of complications such as bleeding and trouble with the anesthesia. After surgery, you are still at risk for infection, discomfort, scar tissue, and problems with healing.

Other problems after breast implant surgery may include your body rejecting the implant, rippling of the skin surface over the implant, and feelings of discomfort and pressure. A capsule of scar tissue can form around the implant, causing it to shrink, feel hard, and sit higher on your rib cage. Additional surgery might be needed to fix it. Breast-feeding is usually still possible after implant surgery (but the effect of the implant on the safety of breast milk is unclear).

When You Want Your Breast Size to Be Different

After breast reduction surgery, healing can take a long time. The scars start out red and bumpy and may take many months to pale. Sometimes the incisions remain red and don't flatten all the way. Complete healing takes time, so it's important to take it easy to get the best results. When the swelling goes away and you reach your final breast size, you may feel very pleased, just okay, or less than happy with your breast size and shape. Future breastfeeding may not be possible.

Emotional Support During and After Breast Surgery

Surgery changes your breast size and shape, but it doesn't automatically change how you think and feel about your breasts, your body, and how you see yourself overall. Feelings of self-consciousness can linger even after surgery. Girls who had very small breasts and got implants could feel just as self-conscious about their new breasts as they did about their old ones. And girls who get reductions may continue to hide in big baggy clothes.

To help take care of all the feelings that can go along with these changes, and to help you adjust to your new breast size, you can benefit from seeing a counselor or therapist. You can ask about sources of emotional support from your doctor or from your school.

If you're not *very* big, *very* small, or *very* uneven, it's much better to solve your breast size change desires with great underwear and stylish clothing. As one girl's mom suggested, "Splurge on the bra, save on the surgery."

Any Questions?

Do breast implants last forever?
Getting breast implants (especially when you're young) means committing

girl to girl

Wow! This is my personal bias, but the fact that breast augmentation is a kind of surgery that needs to be repeated—that just seals the deal for me. Not for me, no thank you. I'm young and my body is still changing. I want to hold on to all my options—including the way-in-the-future idea of nursing.

to multiple surgeries in the future if you want to keep the bigger size. That's because implants usually last about ten to fifteen years. But in someone who is very active they might need to be replaced much sooner. It's not possible to patch the implant, so if it leaks, it has to be replaced. If you change your mind and decide to go back to your original size, you can have both implants removed.

Can liposuction be used to make breasts smaller?

Liposuction (a surgery technique used to remove fat by suctioning it through a tube placed under the skin) is not used to make girls' breasts smaller. This technique may be used in men who want to get rid of unwanted breast enlargement due to extra fat. This procedure is not done in girls because breast fat is mixed in with breast gland tissue, which could be damaged by suction.

How do I pick the size I want to end up being?

Breast surgery for normal-sized breasts is not recommended. It shouldn't be used as a beauty treatment and should only be undertaken after careful consideration of alternatives and possible consequences. Having said that, the best approach to choosing a breast size is to pick what's in proportion to your body. For example, if you are short and stocky, you probably don't want to do an extreme reduction. Or if you are very petite and thin, do not get very large breasts. This stage in the decision-making process requires a careful discussion with your parents, doctors, and nurse-practitioners. Remember too that your breasts will continue to grow and widen until you're in your mid-20s. And they can get bigger with weight gain and smaller with weight loss.

girl to girl

As weird as it is to think that I'll be breast-feeding a baby one day, it's definitely something I would take into consideration seriously if I were considering surgery. For me, wanting to be able to breast-feed a baby is one of those primal instincts I'm glad I haven't lost.

When You Want Your Breast Size to Be Different

Will I be able to breast-feed after breast surgery?
It's important to know that breast reduction surgery will probably take away your ability to breast-feed your baby in the future. So will a breast lift. Breast enlargement with implants *might* affect your ability to do it. (We know that this is unlikely to be an issue for you in your life at this time, but decisions today can affect your life in the future.) While breast-feeding is an extremely personal choice that only you alone will make, doctors strongly believe that breast-feeding is best for your baby and you. Besides the bond it builds between you and your baby, it provides your baby with excellent nutrition and boosts its immune system to fight off infection. Breast-feeding also helps the mom recover from childbirth, burn off calories, and reduce the risk of breast cancer. If you feel strongly about nursing your babies, you might choose to postpone breast reduction surgery until after you are finished having children. All this said, you may feel that breast-feeding may not be right for you or it may seem *sooo* far away from where you are now. You may really want to be able to do it but decide that the burden and physical limitations of having very big breasts today outweigh the benefit of breast feeding in the future. The most important thing is for you to get the facts so you can make a careful choice before you choose surgery.

Does breast surgery increase the risk of breast cancer?
No, surgery to reduce, enlarge, lift, or even out your breasts does not increase your risk of breast cancer. Implants used to enlarge breasts are considered safe and don't increase your risk of cancer or other diseases. But decisions today can impact your future. Implants in a young woman might get in the way of accurate mammography and your ability to breast-feed later on in life.

How much does breast surgery cost? Is it covered by insurance?
The cost of breast surgery depends on the extent of the surgery (one side or both), the use of implants, the anesthesia required, and whether you have to stay in the hospital. It can range from about $6,000 to $8,000 for

basic breast reduction and from about $7,000 to $10,000 (depending on the type of implants) for breast augmentation.

Insurance may cover the cost of surgery if there is a solid medical reason for the surgery. Breast reduction is often covered if your breasts are very large and if you have significant symptoms such as bad posture and shoulder and back problems. Correcting tubular breasts may be covered if they are considered a breast development problem. Making your breasts even may be covered if the difference between your breasts is more than one cup size.

Whatever your situation, a strong letter of support from your plastic surgeon to your medical insurance company is necessary. Also, it's best to get your insurance company to agree to cover the cost before your surgery is done, documented with a letter.

How common is breast surgery done in girls under age 18?
Surgery to make breasts bigger is more common than surgery to make breasts smaller. In 2007, the American Society for Aesthetic Plastic Surgery reported that 7,882 girls age 18 and younger had breast enlargements and 4,207 girls had breast reductions. (Not all breast size surgeries were recorded by this professional group, however.) Compared to about ten years ago, the number of breast enlargements has more than doubled, and the number of reductions has increased by 20 percent.

You can share your stories at TakingCareOfYourGirls.com.

From Tight Bras to Antiperspirants:

Replacing Breast Cancer Fears with Facts

My aunt keeps her money and change in her bra. Once, one of the coins was stuck to her boob. When she was in the shower she felt it, then flipped out because she thought she had cancer.

Erin, 13

It seems like no one really knows what causes breast cancer. It seems like you are at greater risk if it runs in your family. But nowadays people are more aware of it; you can have a mammogram and catch it early.

Kate, 18

I think my grandmother had breast cancer, but no one told me. All of a sudden everyone started giving her pink stuff and she started doing pink ribbon walks. I felt left out and hurt.

Brittany, 19

I was worried about my mom because she had to have an unusual lump in her breast checked out, although it turned out to be a benign cyst.

But I am still a little worried about her because she has had a few more doctor's appointments since then that I think are related, but she hasn't told me about them.

Georgia, 13

My younger sister is always worried about everything, and she was complaining that her breast hurt and she thought she had breast cancer. And she made my mom take her to the doctor and we all knew she didn't have cancer, but she insisted on going only to find out that her breasts were just developing.

Jennifer, 16

My mother came home from a checkup once and told me to be prepared in case anything were to come back showing cancer. Luckily, she didn't have breast cancer, but it was one of the scariest experiences of my life.

Hailey, 17

When I first found out about breast cancer I didn't think it was a big idea, until recently. The breast cancer organization thing is all over the place and it shows me that this is no easy obstacle to overcome. I know a lot of people with breast cancer and now I am worried I will soon get it.

Meredith, 14

My grandmother had breast cancer when she was pregnant with my mother. It was a difficult time because of the medicine she was on and there was the question of whether her baby would be delivered healthy. She had one of her breasts removed. She is now 89 and is a forty-eight-year survivor and is healthier then ever (and my mom is fine).

Annie, 16

I'm always thinking about it because it's always on TV.

Laura, 10

I tried to check my breasts but I got scared because it was a little lumpy. I thought I had breast cancer. But I wouldn't know what normal feels like since I've never compared a cancerous boob to a noncancerous one.

Trish, 12

I remember hearing if you wear a bra to bed, it can contribute to breast cancer. I have also heard that using too much deodorant can also contribute to breast cancer.

Lindsey, 11

First Things First

Breast cancer almost never occurs in girls. But all girls—even those with no one close to them with breast cancer—still worry about the women in their family as well as themselves. About one-third of all middle and high school girls told us that they have already worried at some point that they have had breast cancer. Pink ribbons—the symbol for the fight against breast cancer—are everywhere, even on your cereal box and yogurt. All year long you hear about breast cancer on TV, in magazines, and on the Internet. There are races, walks, and other events in every town and city. Hearing about something scary all the time, no matter what it is, can make anyone feel doomed to get it.

Your worry might have been triggered by feeling a lump in your breast or a shooting pain that keeps coming back. You're also more likely to worry about something you feel in your breast if someone close to you is diagnosed with breast cancer or a celebrity such as Sheryl Crow announces her diagnosis.

Most girls keep their worries a secret. Few girls share their questions and concerns with their mom, doctor, nurse, friend, or other family members. But the best way to resolve your fears and answer your questions is with real, solid information. Knowledge really is power. This chapter will tell you all about breast cancer, addressing facts, feelings, rumors, myths, and concerns.

Here's the Scoop

Breast cancer is *extremely* rare in teens. Nearly all breast cancer occurs in adult women. Over 75 percent of girls 8 to 18 years old say an adult woman close to them has had breast cancer: a mom, grandmother, aunt, neighbor, friend's mom, teacher, coach, or school administrator. The biggest risk factor for getting breast cancer is, in fact, growing older. That means the younger you are, the lower your risk of getting breast cancer; the older you are, the higher the risk. Bottom line: getting breast cancer is *not* something you as a teenager need to worry about. But it is something you need to know about. In this chapter, we're going to help you understand what breast cancer is, its signs and symptoms, who gets it, what you can do about it, and how women who are diagnosed with breast cancer can get well after treatment. You do need to learn how to keep your breasts healthy now, so they can stay healthy over your long, long life ahead.

Breast Cancer is Super-Rare in Girls

As we've said, breast cancer is *very* rare in girls. In fact, most women (88 percent) won't *ever* get breast cancer. But of the cancers that affect women, breast cancer is the most common kind: one in eight women will get breast cancer during her lifetime (that means seven out of eight won't). A bit later we'll tell you about risk factors for breast cancer—the things that make getting breast cancer more or less likely to happen.

What It Is

Breast cancer is an uncontrolled growth of breast cells due to a genetic abnormality. But as we'll explain in the section on risk factors, most of the time the genetic problem does *not* run in a family and cannot be inherited.

All cells inside the breast normally grow and rest, grow and rest,

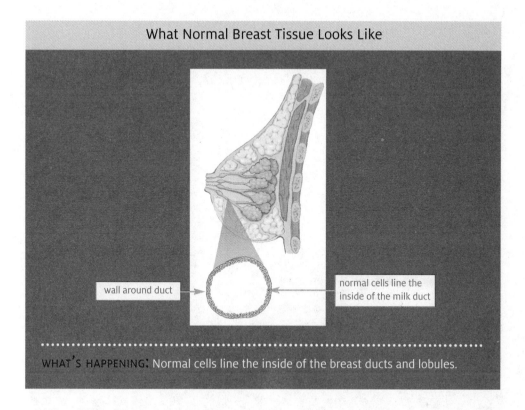

What Normal Breast Tissue Looks Like

wall around duct

normal cells line the inside of the milk duct

WHAT'S HAPPENING: Normal cells line the inside of the breast ducts and lobules.

grow and rest. The illustration above shows you again what the cells normally look like inside the breast lobules (that make milk) and breast ducts (that drain the milk).

The genes inside the breast cells are responsible for controlling the amount of growing and resting that the cells do. If a gene is damaged for whatever reason, it may not be able to do its job properly and an uncontrolled growth of breast cells can result: too much growing, not enough resting. That's what breast cancer is.

When breast cancer first starts, the cells build up and stay inside the breast duct or lobule. That's called *carcinoma in situ*—a fancy way of saying that the cells are still within the place where they started.

Over time, the cancer cells can break out of the breast duct or lobule and invade the surrounding breast tissue, as illustrated on the next

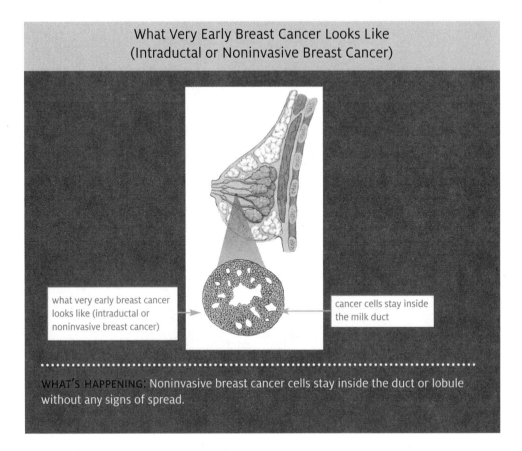

What Very Early Breast Cancer Looks Like
(Intraductal or Noninvasive Breast Cancer)

what very early breast cancer looks like (intraductal or noninvasive breast cancer)

cancer cells stay inside the milk duct

WHAT'S HAPPENING: Noninvasive breast cancer cells stay inside the duct or lobule without any signs of spread.

page. This is called invasive ductal or lobular breast cancer, depending on which part of the breast the cancer cells came from.

As the breast cancer cells grow, they can build up to become a lump or an area of thickening. Sometimes invasive breast cancer cells can spread beyond the breast to lymph nodes nearby and to other parts of the body. (Lymph nodes are an important part of your immune system that help clean the fluid that drains away from the breast.)

Causes of Breast Cancer

Breast cancer is always due to a gene abnormality inside the breast cells. Nine out of ten times, the gene problem that gives rise to a breast

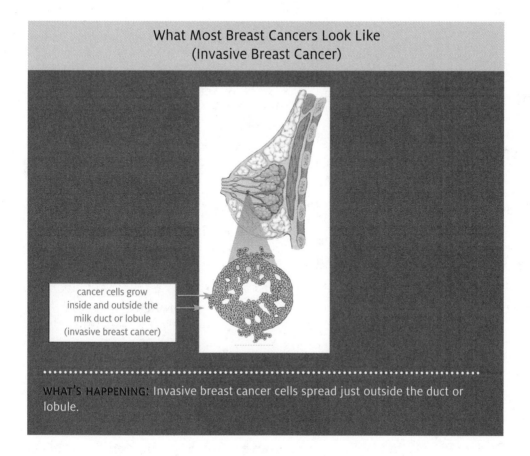

What Most Breast Cancers Look Like
(Invasive Breast Cancer)

cancer cells grow inside and outside the milk duct or lobule (invasive breast cancer)

WHAT'S HAPPENING: Invasive breast cancer cells spread just outside the duct or lobule.

cancer occurs through the wear and tear of living—the aging process. The longer you live, the more wear and tear; that's why the biggest risk factor for breast cancer is growing older. That's also why breast cancer is so rare in girls: because you're so young and you've had very little wear and tear on your genes.

Only one out of ten times does the gene problem run in a family—that's when it's called *inherited*. A breast cancer gene can be passed down from your mom's side or your dad's side of the family.

This means that getting breast cancer usually has nothing to do with having breast cancer in your family. In fact, most women who get breast cancer have no family history of the disease.

Who Gets Breast Cancer and Why

Mature women are the ones who usually get breast cancer. Men can sometimes get breast cancer, but it's very uncommon. It's actually much more likely for men to get breast cancer than young girls—but both are rare.

Even so, all girls want to know: who is most likely to get it and why? Things that might increase a woman's risk of getting breast cancer are called *risk factors.* If you have one or more risk factors, your risk of breast cancer may be higher than that of someone else who is without those risk factors. If you have none of the risk factors, your risk is probably lower than the average person's.

Risk factors come in different sizes. Some of these risk factors are tiny, some are medium, and some are big. Some women have no extra risk factors (besides being a woman and living her life), others have a few small ones, and some women have a bunch of big and small ones. But even if you or someone in your family has a tall stack of risk factors that adds up to something big, it still doesn't mean that you're *going* to get breast cancer. And the opposite is true: women without any extra risk factors could still develop breast cancer. Just for perspective, remember that most women never get breast cancer. And for those who do, it's still very treatable.

There are a lot of rumors spreading around the Internet about things that might increase the risk of getting breast cancer. For example, about 20 percent of girls think breast cancer is caused in part by antiperspirant use, infection, tanning, drug use, stress, or getting bumped in the breast; however, none of these is a risk factor. We're going to review what *are* risk factors for getting breast cancer and what are *not* risk factors. Then later on, in the next chapter, we'll talk about things you can do to improve your breast health and protect yourself against breast cancer. Here are the proven risk factors for breast cancer:

Most Significant Risk Factors

The biggest risk factors for breast cancer are being a woman, growing older, family history, and having a specific type of genetic abnormality (usually called the "breast cancer gene") in the family. Having had breast cancer in the past also puts you at higher risk for getting it in the future.

- **BEING A WOMAN.** Breast cancer is much more common in women than in men. Each year in the USA, about 240,000 women are diagnosed with breast cancer compared to 2,000 men.

- **GROWING OLDER.** As women grow older, their risk of breast cancer goes up. When you are very, very young, your risk of getting breast cancer is very, very low. Older women have the higher risk.

- **FAMILY HISTORY OF BREAST CANCER.** The risk of breast cancer in women who have family members with breast cancer depends on a lot of things, including how many women and men have had it and at what age, and if there are other kinds of cancer in the family, such as ovarian cancer, colon cancer, and thyroid cancer. Families with a strong history of breast cancer (and some of these other cancers) may choose to be tested for the gene abnormality.

- **GENETIC ABNORMALITY.** About 10 percent of breast cancers (one out of ten cases of breast cancer) are due to an inherited breast cancer gene abnormality that runs in a family. Many families with a breast cancer gene abnormality also have a strong family history of breast cancer.

girl to girl

Wow wow wow! Hold up. How is it that the two biggest risk factors are things we have no control over? Being a woman and growing older are supposed to be exciting, not scary, right? Of course! What we do have control over is how we take care of ourselves.

- **PERSONAL HISTORY OF BREAST CANCER.** If a woman has had breast cancer once in her life, she may be at a higher risk of getting another breast cancer in the future. That's different from recurrence, which is the return of a prior cancer. Chances are she won't get breast cancer again, either a recurrence or a new one, but she needs to be more careful than the average person.

Small to Medium-Sized Risk Factors

Next is a bunch of small to medium-sized risk factors for breast cancer that—one way or another—involve hormones. Estrogen and other hormones can get the breast cells all jazzed up. A higher than normal level of hormones for a long period of time can turn on regular breast cell growth, and occasionally promote cancer cell growth.

- **THE LONGER YOU MENSTRUATE.** Starting your period at an early age (before age 12) and stopping your period late (after age 55) usually means that your body sees a higher level of hormones for a longer chunk of time. Long-term hormonal stimulation can give breast cells the wrong idea—to misbehave and possibly start a cancer. This is a small risk factor.

- **NO FULL-TERM PREGNANCY OR FIRST FULL-TERM PREGNANCY AFTER AGE 30 OR NO BREAST-FEEDING.** It's healthy for breasts to have a break in the usual hormonal action. A full-term pregnancy and breast-feeding bring on a change of hormonal "scenery" and put some strict new rules of behavior in place, forcing breast cells to get their act together, mature, get a job (get ready to make milk), and report to work (start making the milk). When the breast cells are so preoccupied with doing the important job of nourishing a baby, they have less time to do things like starting a cancer. (A miscarriage or abortion does not seem to make breast cancer risk go up or down—the important new job wasn't in place long enough to have a benefit.) This is a small risk factor. These factors can also balance and cancel each other out. For example, if you had your first baby at age 30 but you breast-fed for nine months, the benefit of breast-feeding can take away some of the risk of a later first pregnancy.

- **HORMONE THERAPY AFTER MENOPAUSE.** Later on in life, your hormonal levels drop and your periods stop—a time called menopause. Unpleasant symptoms can occur due to the lower hormone levels. To feel better, some women take hormone medication. But keeping hormone levels up over time can lead to a slightly higher risk of breast cancer.

- **BEING OVERWEIGHT.** Extra fat starts breast growth earlier and makes a bunch of extra hormones. Over time, these hormones can overstimulate the breast cells, leading to a higher risk of breast cancer. This is a small to medium risk factor, depending on the amount of extra weight. Fat can also store trouble-making chemicals and hormones from the environment.

- **HORMONES IN FOOD AND DRINKS.** Very low levels of hormones or chemicals that can behave like hormones can get into our food and drinks. For example, a small amount of pesticide, used to keep the bugs off growing plants, can stick to or get inside the fruit and vegetables that you eat. Another example is a hormone-like chemical in hard plastic water bottles that can leach into your drinks. Hormones given to cows to increase their milk supply can get into their milk. Hormones given to animals to make them bigger can get into their meat and be stored in their fat. So foods that have high levels of animal fat, such as red meat and ice cream, can contain these hormones. Eating or drinking these low levels of hormones and hormone-like substances over long periods of time might stimulate breast cells and could cause trouble. The size of this risk factor is not known, but it is probably small, depending on a lot of factors that will be discussed further in Chapter 12.

- **ALCOHOL.** Drinking alcohol on a regular basis over the years can lead to a slightly higher risk of breast cancer. Your liver has to work overtime to get rid of the alcohol, and as a result, it neglects its regular job to lower the hormone levels in your blood. As a result, hormone levels stay higher than they're supposed to. Also, alcohol can lead to weight gain because it has a lot of calories. Then the extra weight can make extra hormones that are not breast-healthy. This is a small to medium risk factor, depending on how much alcohol is consumed.

- **LITTLE PHYSICAL ACTIVITY.** Being physically inactive is a risk factor for breast cancer. It's partly because you tend to weigh more when you're inactive. On the flip side, when you exercise you tend to make a lot of other healthy choices, such as managing your weight, eating well, not smoking, and limiting alcohol use.

There are other small risk factors with no clear explanation for why or how they can increase breast cancer risk.

- SMOKING. Of course, smoking is unhealthy for many, many reasons, including increasing breast cancer risk. Besides damaging your lungs, the nicotine in cigarettes is a poison to your body. It narrows all of your little blood vessels, making it harder to flush out the fluids, hormones, and other chemicals in your breasts that are normally quickly cleared from your body. This kind of chemical buildup can damage your breast cells. People who smoke are also more likely to do other unhealthy things such as drink a lot of alcohol and avoid physical activity.

- CHARCOAL-GRILLED, HIGH-FAT, OR FRIED FOODS. Research shows a small connection between eating large amounts of these foods over time and a small increase in the risk of breast cancer.

Not Risk Factors

There are tons of rumors and myths floating around about what causes breast cancer. The following things have *no* proven influence on breast cancer risk:

- THINGS YOU WEAR OR USE. Wearing a regular or underwire bra during the day or night and wearing tight clothing do not affect breast cancer risk. Using antiperspirants, deodorants, or a cell phone does not increase the risk of breast cancer. Neither does coffee or chocolate. Today's birth control pills have no clear connection to breast cancer risk; however, none of today's many new birth control pills have been studied long enough to know their breast health safety. Studies based on old-fashioned pills that contained relatively higher amounts of hormones showed at most a small increased risk that disappeared after the pills were stopped. Most doctors believe that current birth control pills do not have a significant influence on breast cancer

girl to girl

Being at risk for breast cancer doesn't mean you're going to get it. Women on both my mother and father's side of the family have breast cancer. It makes me a little nervous, but not scared. I can't change who my family is, but I can change what I do each day. Most days I'm pretty good about doing the right things. But sometimes I'm lazy, too tired, or too busy, and things slip. That's okay. I'm certainly not perfect. I just try to do the best that I can.

risk. Talk with your doctor if you are considering taking birth control pills and weigh the benefits and side effects for your specific situation.

- **THINGS YOU MIGHT DO.** Sunbathing and tanning are bad for your skin and can increase your risk of skin cancer, but they have no effect on breast cancer risk. Using drugs is unhealthy for you in many ways, as you well know. But drug use has no effect on breast cancer risk.

- **THINGS THAT MIGHT HAPPEN TO YOU.** Stress in your life makes you feel bad, but it doesn't change your risk of breast cancer on its own. If stress makes you smoke, drink alcohol, stop exercising, or eat too much and gain weight, then it can indirectly increase your risk. Getting a bump, a bruise, or an infection in your breast does not increase your risk. Touching or fondling does not increase the risk of breast cancer.

> ### girl to girl
>
> I was at a sleepover birthday party in seventh grade with about twenty or so girls from my class. We were all sitting around talking, and one of the girls, someone who we all particularly trusted and respected, said that it was clinically proven that wearing a bra overnight causes breast cancer. As soon as I got home the next day I asked my mom if it was true. She said absolutely not!

Keep in mind: being at risk for something does *not* necessarily mean it's going to happen! It just means that you need to make a bigger effort to lead a healthy life, check yourself more carefully and regularly, and work more closely with your doctors to stay well and productive. All of these healthy steps are addressed in Chapter 12.

Even though your risk of breast cancer is slight, most girls feel better knowing just exactly how adult women discover and treat their breast cancer.

How Breast Cancer Is Discovered

Signs and Symptoms

All girls want to know: what are the signs (something that you notice) and symptoms (a new feeling that you become aware of) of breast cancer? But before we review them with you, it's important for you to know two big things:

- NONE OF THE FOLLOWING SIGNS AND SYMPTOMS IS UNIQUE TO BREAST CANCER. The most common sign, feeling a lump in your breast, is much, much more likely to be normal than it is to be from cancer. Breast redness is much, much more likely to be from an infection or rash than from cancer. Breast pain is also much, much more likely to be due to a normal cause than from cancer. So don't freak out as we go through this list, since most of the time having one or more of these signs or symptoms does *not* mean you have cancer.

- NEARLY ALL OF THE INFORMATION IN THIS SECTION ABOUT BREAST CANCER SIGNS, SYMPTOMS, DETECTION, TREATMENT, AND RECOVERY IS BASED ON OLDER WOMEN. In fact, the average age of a woman diagnosed with breast cancer is about 60. And because breast cancer is so rare in girls, there are almost no studies of girls with breast cancer.

Most breast cancers in adult women are found by feeling a lump or seeing an abnormality on a mammogram (a picture of the breasts). Breast cancer may also be found by other kinds of tests besides mammography, such as an ultrasound or MRI.

Here are some of the signs of breast cancer:

- A LUMP IN THE BREAST OR UNDER THE ARM. A woman or her doctor might notice a lump in her breast that feels firm or hard, doesn't go away, or gets bigger. Sometimes a lump can show up in an armpit lymph node from cancer cells that spread from the breast. But, again, most lumps are *not* cancer.

- A THICKENING IN THE BREAST. Occasionally, cancer can feel like a thick area of tissue in the breast (not anything round)—sort of like an area of stiff carpeting, surrounded by a regular plush shag carpet with a lot of padding.

- A CHANGE IN THE SHAPE OR SIZE OF THE BREAST. Sometimes the breast can look different on the outside. A woman might notice a bulge, dimple, or dent. Or perhaps part or all of the breast appears bigger. A nipple that used to point out might flatten and tuck inside. As breast cancer grows, it pulls in tissue around it, and that's how it changes the shape of the breast.

- **REDNESS OR A RASH.** Occasionally, a change in the color of the breast could be a sign of breast cancer. A relatively rare form of breast cancer involves redness and swelling of part or all of the breast.

- **A SORE ON THE BREAST.** Very occasionally, a sore might develop on the surface of the breast or nipple/areola that might itch, bleed, and refuse to heal or go away. It might even get bigger. There could be a lump right underneath the sore spot that feels a little like a mosquito bite. When this happens, only rarely is it a breast cancer. Much more commonly it's acne or a real bug bite that you may have scratched and it got irritated or infected.

- **NIPPLE DISCHARGE.** If blood comes out of one nipple, it's usually not cancer. It usually comes from a bunch of normal cells hanging out in the milk pipe under the nipple. In girls, it's rarely a sign of a breast cancer growth underneath.

Most of the time, breast cancer causes no symptoms—no pain, itching, throbbing, or other feelings. But if there are new and unusual symptoms in one breast that don't go away or that get worse, if they are different from period-related breast symptoms, and if your instincts tell you that something's not right, then let your doctor know. It's *very* unlikely that it will be breast cancer, but it's still important to check things out.

Tests

Most breast cancers are found through routine tests done for the purpose of early detection in women age 40 and older who have no breast signs or symptoms. The routine tests we're talking about are the ones described in Chapter 3: mammograms, your doctor's physical examination, and your own breast self-examination.

Tests may be done in women who develop new breast signs or symptoms that don't go away or get worse. An ultrasound, mammogram, and sometimes an MRI are done. Sometimes a biopsy will be done to check out a piece of the tissue with a microscope. If test results show that there is a breast cancer present, then additional studies are done to figure out the situation and determine what treatments are needed. Learning about the nature and extent of the problem is accomplished by a bunch of tests, such as the pathology report, a mammogram, ultrasound, MRI scan, blood tests, and more.

Understanding the Cancer

After a breast cancer has been discovered, doctors work to figure out the nature of the problem. This is done with laboratory tests that look at how fast it's growing, the presence of any gene abnormalities, its response to hormones, and if there are cancer cells in the fluid channels of the breasts.

After doctors understand the nature of the breast cancer, next they figure out its stage, based on the size of the cancer in the breast and if there is any spread to lymph nodes and other parts of the body.

Once both the nature and stage have been figured out, a treatment plan is designed to get rid of the cancer. Each person gets a treatment plan that's tailored to her unique situation. That's why one woman's treatment can be very different from another's.

How Breast Cancer Is Treated

No matter what kind or stage of cancer a woman might have, there are effective therapies that can be given to get rid of the cancer or keep it under control.

Every cancer, even the very small ones, is made up of different kinds of breast cancer cells. This is the reason why different forms of treatment (radiation, surgery, various chemotherapies, hormonal therapy), which work in different ways, are usually given to get rid of the different types of cells that are in one cancer.

There are two main kinds of breast cancer treatment: local therapies and systemic therapies. Local treatment focuses on the breast and nearby lymph nodes using surgery and sometimes radiation. Systemic treatment addresses the whole body (or system) with medicine.

Local treatment usually treats the whole breast (and some lymph nodes too) one way or another.

- **Mastectomy** is a surgery to remove the whole breast. Sometimes women need to have a mastectomy because the cancer is large or there is more than one cancer in the same breast.

- **Lumpectomy** is a surgery to remove the cancer from the breast. The rest of the breast remains in place after the surgery.

- **Radiation** is an anticancer treatment that uses high-energy rays or particles, produced by a machine or by placing radiation-emitting material directly into the area of concern.

Breast preservation therapy is a combination of lumpectomy and radiation. Surgery can remove the cancer, and then radiation is used to treat the rest of the breast. A new approach to treating the breast is partial breast treatment—that's when the lump is removed and radiation is given only to the area around where the cancer was.

Systemic therapy involves medicines that are given by pill or through the bloodstream (using an IV).

> ## girl to girl
>
> The summer after my grandma was diagnosed with breast cancer, it really hit me. We're always on the beach together, so after her mastectomy, you could really see that she had had breast cancer because her breast is missing. It was a little weird at first, but then I began to think of it as her battle scar—a battle that, thankfully, she won.

- **Chemotherapy** involves special chemicals that are designed to get rid of cancer cells. Since the treatment is delivered to the entire body, normal cells are also affected. That's why most women going through chemotherapy lose their hair: the same chemicals fighting the cancer also affect the cells that make hair.

- **Hormonal therapy** stops hormones from turning on breast cancer cells that need hormones for their growth.

- **Targeted therapies** are designed to get rid of the cancer cells and leave the normal cells alone. The treatment is aimed at a specific gene or protein that's only or mostly in the cancer cells and not present in normal tissue. A medicine named Herceptin is the best known targeted therapy. The goal is to provide effective anticancer therapy and avoid side effects.

Complementary medicine supports the whole person—her mind and her body—along with the cancer-fighting treatments described above. It can help improve a person's energy, nutrition, movement, relaxation, and immune system, as well as decrease side effects of treatment or cancer, such as pain and fatigue. Types of complementary therapies that you might have heard of include meditation, massage, special diets, and yoga. Emotional support through online communities (www.breastcancer.org has tons of them), support groups, and individual therapy is also really important.

To get the best possible treatment plan, a woman dealing with breast cancer usually works with a team of doctors who are experts in all areas of cancer treatment. What treatment comes first, next, and last is tailored to each patient.

There are some women who have cancer that has spread beyond the breast and lymph nodes. This is called *metastatic* breast cancer. Medicine therapy is the main form of treatment

girl to girl

My mom has taken care of women with breast cancer for twenty years and she started two nonprofits in our house (they're in regular offices now). So for my whole life, I've been surrounded by so many brave women who have fought the battle against breast cancer. So many seem to win the battle. There are some women who are in an ongoing battle and continue to lead pretty full lives. But, as incredible as today's medicine is, the battle against breast cancer is sometimes lost. Some of the strongest, most amazing women I've ever known have been patients of my mom who have died. It's one of the hardest things to come to terms with, but it's just one of those very tough things in life that isn't fair. Instead of dwelling on the loss for too long, my mom and I celebrate the lives of these special women lost to breast cancer, and we keep up a special relationship with their families. Our book is dedicated to their memory.

used. Surgery and radiation can also be used if there is a specific concern that needs addressing.

After treatment is over, it's very important that women take time to heal and recover. Over time, they will feel better and more like themselves. But all along the way to recovery, they can get stronger and stay determined to enjoy each day, become as healthy as possible, and remain cancer-free.

Any Questions?

Breast cancer runs in my family—does that mean I'm going to get it?
Even if women in your family have the inherited kind of breast cancer, it doesn't mean that you will automatically get it. Your risk may or may not be increased.

If your mother or father carries a breast cancer gene, you have a 50 percent chance of *not* getting that gene, in which case your risk would be just like any other girl or woman. But you also have a 50 percent risk of getting the gene. However, even if you did get the gene, it's not at all certain that you'd get breast cancer. There's a 40–85 percent risk spread out over a lifetime, depending on the type of gene, the way the gene behaves in your particular family, the way you live your life, and the environment that surrounds you.

You can read more about breast cancer and genes at:
www.breastcancer.org.

Does having a family history of breast cancer mean getting it earlier in life (although my mom and grandmom were older)?
Families with a lot of women with breast cancer or a known breast cancer gene do tend to get breast cancer at younger ages than other women without this background. But it's still very rare to get it as a teenager or in your early 20s. Your mom and grandmother's breast cancer may or may not impact your risk of getting breast cancer. When you're older, like over age 18, you can discuss this further with a genetics

counselor to learn more about your family's risk. In the meantime, you can, like every girl and woman, learn how to become as healthy as possible (see Chapter 12).

Is breast cancer that runs in a family more serious?
It's important to know that breast cancer that runs in families is no more serious than the much more common noninherited type. But what is true of inherited breast cancer is that the risk of developing a separate, new breast cancer in the future is higher (different from a recurrence, which is when the prior breast cancer returns). This would mean that your family members have to be extra careful taking care of themselves, following *extra* steps to reduce their risk of getting breast cancer.

What are the types of breast cancer genes?
The two most common inherited types of breast cancer genes are named BRCA1 and BRCA2 (*BRCA* stands for "breast cancer"). If a mother or father has one of these genes, their children have equal chances of *not* getting the gene and of getting the gene. But even getting the gene doesn't automatically mean you're definitely going to develop cancer. A genetic counselor can work with your family to provide valuable information and testing.

What is the most common age to get breast cancer?
The average age of a woman getting breast cancer is 60. About 25 percent of breast cancers occur in women under age 50. The rest, 75 percent, happen after age 50.

Do only women get breast cancer?
Both women and men get breast cancer, although it is much more common in women. That's because women's breasts are developed and active, whereas men's breasts usually don't develop and the tissues inside them are inactive. (When you see a man with big breasts, it's usually because of extra fat rather than from extra breast tissue.)

From Tight Bras to Antiperspirants

Why do some people survive breast cancer and some don't? Isn't it all the same cancer?
Most women survive breast cancer when cancer is found in its early stages. But there are some types of breast cancer that are harder to treat and get rid of or keep under control. No two cancers are the same. The nature of each breast cancer is unique. That's why doctors spend so much time in the beginning trying to figure out exactly what kind of breast cancer is present. If the nature of the cancer seems to be fast growing and aggressive, then stronger treatments will be required to effectively fight back.

What happens if you don't get treated?
If breast cancer is present and no treatment is given, the cancer will grow. It's very important to get the most effective treatment possible in order to eliminate the cancer or keep it from growing.

It could grow slowly or quickly, depending on the nature and extent of the cancer. When a breast cancer is first discovered, it takes time to figure these things out. Treatment isn't started until the best plan can be made. That's okay—it's much more important to take the time to make the best treatment plan than it is to rush into treatment.

What happens if cancer comes back?
Sometimes, even after very good treatment, cancer may return. If that happens, the doctors work hard with the patient to figure out the extent and the nature of the new situation. Tests are done and new therapy options are evaluated. A whole new treatment plan is designed. There are a lot of reasons to believe and hope that the cancer can be gotten rid of or put under control.

Is it your own fault that you get breast cancer?
No! Getting breast cancer does *not* mean that the person or anyone else did anything wrong! Sins don't lead to breast cancer. And kids who get in a lot of trouble don't increase their mother's risk (nor their own risk) of getting breast cancer.

When a diagnosis of breast cancer occurs, no one should think it was her fault. Instead, people in her life should help the patient feel good about herself and give her the strength and support she needs to deal with her situation, get through treatment, and fully recover. It's also important to take the opportunity to follow a healthy lifestyle and diet to reduce the risk of cancer in the future.

Can you get breast cancer if you've had breast augmentation or breast reduction surgery?
Breast cancer can still happen. These surgery procedures have no impact on breast cancer risk.

Do breast implants hide lumps?
Implants appear completely white on a mammogram. You cannot see through them. Special techniques are needed to see all of the breast tissue around the implant. Usually all of the breast tissue can be seen. But it is possible that small areas of the breast are hard to see. If there is a lump in that hard-to-see spot, then it might be hidden. MRI and ultrasound tests are usually able to see around the implant without any problem.

If you get breast cancer when you're pregnant, can you pass it to your child?
If a mother has cancer, the cancer cells cannot pass from the mother into the baby. They would be stopped by the placenta, where the mom's blood delivers nutrients and picks up waste products from the baby. If a mom has a breast cancer gene, there is a 50 percent risk that the baby will get the gene.

If you have breast cancer and are treated, are you still able to breast-feed?
After breast cancer treatment, the breast that had the cancer in it is usually unable to make milk. If the breast was removed with or without reconstruction, it cannot make milk. After partial breast removal and radiation, breast-feeding in that breast is unlikely. But the other side

usually works just fine, and it can usually produce enough milk to feed a baby. If not, the mom might need to use some bottle feedings in addition to her own breast milk. Also, the baby cannot get breast cancer from breast milk.

Is it true that everyone has a small amount of cancer in their bodies, but only some grow?
No. Everyone's cells are growing and resting every day and night. It's not uncommon for a group of cells to misbehave and grow a little out of control. But your body is usually pretty quick to step in and get things back under control. Most extra cell growth is not cancer and won't become cancer.

Is there a relationship between breast size and the occurrence of breast cancer?
No. The size of your breasts has no influence on your risk of breast cancer. Big breasts and small breasts have the same risk.

What is the risk of getting breast cancer more than once?
There are many things that can predict the risk of getting breast cancer again in the future. A return of the original breast cancer is called a recurrence. The start of a new cancer, in either breast, can also happen. The risk of recurrence or a new cancer depends on the nature of the first cancer, the effectiveness of the treatment, and a bunch of other risk factors, such as if there is a breast cancer gene in the family.

Do some ethnic groups get breast cancer more than others?
The risk factors described above are much more significant than the effect of ethnic or racial background on a woman's risk of breast cancer. In countries where women tend to be slim, physically active, don't smoke, and have a diet of mostly fruits and vegetables—like Japan or China—their risk of breast cancer is relatively low. In the United States, white women are more likely to get breast cancer than African American women overall—but in women under age 40, it's more common in

African Americans. Jewish women originally from Eastern Europe have a higher risk. As more ethnic groups intermingle and as lifestyles change, many of these differences can change and even disappear.

Does your body type put you at greater risk?
Bodies come in all different shapes and sizes. Bodies that are apple-shaped (bigger in the middle belly area) seem to have a higher risk of breast cancer than bodies that are pear-shaped (bigger in the hips and rear end). It's not clear exactly why, but it probably has to do with the extra hormones made by belly fat which can turn on breast cell activity. Of course, you can't change the kind of body that you have, but through exercise and weight management, you can definitely become very healthy.

Reading about breast cancer makes me worried. How do I deal with that?
This chapter may have given you lots of extra things to worry about when you think about your breasts. If what you've read applies to you, you have ways to deal with the issues. If you are without any breast cancer concerns, then think of this chapter as a health lesson. But maybe you know someone who has an issue that's been described—now you can be an understanding and helpful friend. Accurate facts are always a valuable gift, especially when there is something positive you can do with that information.

Use this information for yourself or pass it along to all the women you care about: your mom, grandmother, friend, neighbor, or teacher. Or you can share it in class or use it for a health assignment. When you share health information with someone else, that's a community service—and you can also go to our nonprofit organization's Web site, www.breastcancer.org, to learn about our community service program.

No one in my family has had breast cancer—does that mean I'm safe?
Every girl and woman needs to care about breast health. Family history is only one of the risk factors. As we discussed in this chapter, being a

woman and growing older are the biggest risk factors. In fact, most women who get breast cancer have no family history of the disease.

How can I help my mom as she goes through breast cancer treatment?
It is very hard for a daughter to see her mom going through breast cancer. First, the most important way to take care of your mom is to be sure to take care of yourself. Eat properly, get good sleep, ask questions, share your feelings and fears, and find out what to expect. Another important way you can help your mom is by spending some time with her and asking her how she is feeling. Plus, the whole family can help by pitching in around the house without being asked: make dinner, set and clear the table, load and unload the dishwasher, do laundry, run errands. You will see how all of these things can make a very big difference and can mean so much to your mom.

You can share your stories at TakingCareOfYourGirls.com.

I want to do everything I can to keep my "puppies" healthy and happy—and never let anything not-so-good come near them.

Michelle, 16

Think Pink, Live Green:

A Planet-Friendly Guide for Healthy Breasts

There's a lot you can do to make sure you're healthy, and it's really important now that you're growing up and developing.

Ivy, 19

I'm willing to change my ways and eat much better than I do as long as it's easy and doesn't cut into my allowance.

Jasmine, 13

Right after health class at school is my lunch block. Exactly what the class says we shouldn't eat is all that's available on the school cafeteria's lunch menu.

Maddie, 15

Gym class has been cut back to once a week and all the non-varsity teams were cut, too. And the exercise room is now closed after school. Now I never get a chance to exercise.

Chelsea, 12

Just after our school ran a special fund-raiser selling plastic water bottles with our logo on it, they took them back because of a "safety problem." Everyone got their money back. Now I just buy my water from the soda machine.

Bianca, 13

I would like to know if there are any ways I could decrease my chance of getting breast cancer.

Amy, 10

My dad got on this big health kick and now most of the food around the house has no taste, looks gross, and has a weird texture. My friends don't like eating over anymore. Now we go out to eat or I go to their house.

Akili, 19

I'm totally confused. One day they say that beans are all good. The next day chocolate, coffee, and soybeans are out. A few months later, dark chocolate is back in. Why can't they agree on this stuff? It's not like these foods are new.

Mary Kate, 17

What's worse: gaining weight from regular sodas or the fake sweeteners in diet soda?

Donna, 15

My parents give mixed messages all the time. At home we have to eat super-healthy, but as soon as we go out, everyone gets to order whatever they want within a certain price range (with no health guidelines).

Patty, 17

First Things First

You can do many things every day at home, in school, and around your community to keep your breasts healthy as well as improve your overall health and peace of mind. And it turns out that the same things that are healthy for your breasts are often better for the environment: walking instead of driving; drinking filtered tap water, not bottled water; stopping smoking; and eating organic foods without pesticides, hormones, preservatives, or artificial fertilizers. With fewer chemicals going into our food and water supply, less smoke in the air, and fewer plastics being used, the world environment becomes healthier for everyone. Thus, you can see how the external environment in which we live is tightly and continuously blended with and affecting the internal environment within our bodies.

In this chapter we want to look at all the different ways to increase your breast health, reduce the risk of breast cancer, and keep the planet healthy, too. The breast-healthy steps that you have the most control over are your physical activity level, your weight, the foods you eat, the water and beverages you drink, and the personal products you use. As you can imagine, anything you do to or put into or onto your body can be helpful, harmless, or harmful. You want to make sure that you and your family make the healthiest choices.

There are things you and your family can start right away. From Chapter II, you know about the risk factors for breast cancer: ones you can't change, ones you can change a little, and some that you can change a lot. We're going to help you address those that you can change. Then we'll talk about extra steps you can take to be as healthy as possible. We want to be completely up front with you: it's going to take daily commitment and effort to have healthy breasts. It's impossible to do everything right 100 percent of the time. We all have to try, though, and give ourselves credit for our dedication and hard work along the way.

One more thing before we move ahead with this chapter: being healthy requires cooperation from your family or your immediate support network. Some of the things we will talk to you about involve things that you might have little control over, such as buying and cooking food. That's okay. This might be a good time to share this book with your family. You can get more done and have more fun when you do these things together.

Here's the Scoop

Let's first take the proven risk factors for breast cancer. If you can take the things that make the risk go up and change them, then you can reduce your risk and increase your breast health. You want to be open to all of the healthy changes you can make, from lifestyle changes to medical therapies.

While it's true that you can't change risk factors such as being a woman, growing older, family history, having a breast cancer gene in the family, and personal history of breast cancer, there are other risk factors you can change.

The good news is you can make a big difference in your breast health. You can make some big risk factors much smaller and you can make some small risks go away. Yes, it definitely takes work—we never said it would be effortless. But think about it: most good things in life take work, effort, and determination. You have to start somewhere, tackle one thing at a time, and put good habits in place. When you do, you'll be rewarded by feeling better, looking better, and feeling the pride that you're taking care of your greatest gift: your life.

No Smoking

Smoking is terrible for your health and leads to a higher risk of breast cancer. The best thing is never to start smoking. The next best thing is to stop. And along with that, avoid or minimize secondhand smoke (when you breathe in other people's smoke). If a family member smokes, approach him or her with a plan that considers the health of everyone in the household. Ask if you can apply the same kind of rules that many businesses have in place: a smoke-free environment. If the person needs to smoke, then ask him or her to go outside and stay away from the front door. Kids are more likely to get their parents or relatives to stop smoking than one of their parents' peers are.

If your friends smoke, it's easier to figure out healthy ways for you to hang out together than it is to find a new group of nonsmoking friends. Take public transportation to avoid driving in a car (where they are more likely to smoke). And if you do drive around together, ask them not to smoke in the car. If it's their car and they're doing you a favor by giving you a ride, you can still ask them politely to open their window. You can also sit next to another car window and open that. Cross ventilation makes a big difference.

Whenever possible, meet your smoking friends outside, not in a closed-in space. Doing a physical activity with a smoking friend, like going running or to the gym, makes it unlikely that they will smoke during that visit. Or meet at places where smoking is not allowed: a restaurant, bookstore café, or mall. Of course, you can also work on your good friends to stop smoking; that's a powerful part of loving someone. Offer to help them in any way you can, like going to a quit-smoking meeting or helping to set a cigarette limit.

No Drinking, Smart Thinking

To reduce your risk of breast cancer, we recommend that you follow the United States law: no drinking alcohol until you're age 21. After age 21, limit your use of alcohol to fewer than five drinks a week. Less is better. Any kind of alcohol counts the same toward breast cancer risk: beer, wine, and hard liquors such as vodka and gin.

The other breast-healthy reason to avoid or limit the use of alcohol is for better nutrition and weight management. You want to avoid the high number of empty calories in alcoholic beverages: one can of beer is about 120 calories, a glass of wine is 90 calories, and a four-ounce daiquiri is about 220 calories (see www.calorie-count.com). You also want to avoid over-eating the high calorie foods that often go along with drinking, like French fries, potato chips, pizza, cheese steaks, and nachos as well as sugary foods like cookies and candy. Drinking combined with these calorie-heavy foods is unhealthy and can add to weight gain.

Sticking to a Healthy Weight

When you're a little kid, is seems as though you can eat whatever you want and never gain an ounce. But after puberty, that can change. The process in which your body converts the food you eat into useful energy is called *metabolism*. When you're little, your metabolism is really fast—meaning that your food is converted to energy quickly and has no time to turn into fat. As you get older, your metabolism slows and more of the food you eat is kept in storage as fat. A certain amount of fat on your body is healthy, but too much or too little can cause you to be over- or underweight.

Getting to and sticking with a healthy weight to keep your breasts healthy requires eating well and staying physically active.

Start with a reality check: visit your doctor, nurse practitioner, or school nurse to find out what your weight is now and what a healthy weight would be for your height and body type. If you're already at a healthy weight, use these tips to help maintain it. If you're under- or overweight, let that healthy weight be your goal. Promise that you'll be nice to yourself and be your own cheerleader. If you start being too self-critical, you can get your weight management off track. You have to support yourself if you're going to make progress.

girl to girl

Because I'm tall, my ideal body weight has always been higher than the rest of my friends'. For a while, I was self-conscious because all my friends always weighed less than me. I was horrified when I was one of the first girls to break 100 pounds in middle school! Looking back, I was silly to think I was overweight—I was just the right weight for my proportion and body type. And all girls gain weight during puberty as you grow up and fill out—it's natural, normal, and healthy.

Talk to your doctor or nutritionist about a diet plan that works best for you. What keeps you motivated? Maybe it's the thought of bikini weather fast approaching or wanting to keep fitting into your favorite jeans. Whatever your personal motivation, find it and stick with it.

Instead of diet shakes, powders, processed foods, and diet pills, many of which contain extra sweeteners, oils, and artificial ingredients, eat a balanced diet of healthy food. Food tastes good when it contains fat, sugar, and salt, but when healthy foods are processed with these ingredients—like when an apple and oatmeal become an apple granola snack bar—the calorie count shoots up and the nutritional value falls down. You'd be much better off with the whole, unprocessed foods.

Physical Activity and Regular Exercise

Physical activity is breast-healthy, as well as a critical part of weight management. You need energy to be active, and exercise is a good way to speed up your metabolism and burn calories from the storage of fat. Diet alone and exercise alone are hard ways to control your weight. But together, they work hand in hand to maintain a healthy weight.

It's best to get in the habit of exercising regularly. Set an exercise goal of 30 minutes a day, or a total of three and a half hours or more per week. Of course, school sports count too. Mix it up—find several types of exercise that get all your muscles moving, your heart pumping, and your lungs breathing faster. Pick the kinds of things you're likely to keep doing over

girl to girl

The coach asked the soccer team who wanted to be the goalie; no one said anything. I didn't want the team to be without a goalie, so I volunteered to do it. It wasn't as fun as I thought it would be! I was stuck standing in front of the net, dressed from head to toe in pads, sweating but not getting any exercise. Everyone else was running around the field. I was unhappy and my mother was unhappy. Our family has a long history of breast cancer and it has always been really important to exercise regularly. So my mom helped me talk to the coach and we ended up taking turns at the position.

time: walking, going to the gym, biking, spinning, swimming, step aerobics, Pilates, or yoga. Your leg and butt muscles are the biggest—make sure to work those babies to burn energy and get into shape the fastest.

Hormone Medications

You can help keep your breasts healthy and reduce the risk of breast cancer by not putting extra hormones into your body that can increase breast cell growth. That's why hormone therapy after menopause (when menstrual periods end, around age 50) is discouraged.

Birth control medicine replaces your regular hormones and takes charge of your menstrual cycle (like a substitute teacher). As long as the medicine doesn't increase your normal hormone levels or make your breasts a lot bigger, then your breast tissue is probably not being over-stimulated and there should be no increased risk of breast cancer.

Pregnancy and Breast-feeding

Having a baby lowers your risk of breast cancer. Pregnancy before age 30 protects your breasts a little bit more than after age 30, but having a baby at any age is still protective. Later in life, when you are ready and if you choose to become a parent and start a family, you may want to consider this factor. And after you have a baby, breast-feeding is important not only for your breast health but also for the health of your baby.

Balancing Your Diet

A breast-healthy diet is low in fat and balanced by a rich mix of all food groups: fruits, vegetables, grains, fish, meat, poultry, and dairy products. Few fast foods meet the mark. It's best to prepare, cook, store, and carry around your food in healthy ways. You want to enjoy your food, eat enough to give your body the energy and nutrients it needs, and avoid overeating. In the next few sections, we'll go over each food group and the best ways to bring them together to be nourished by them.

Food: What's Good and Good for You

Of course you want foods with the most nutrients and the least amount of unhealthy chemicals. In the food-growing world, various chemicals are used to:

- Keep the bugs and fungus off (pesticides, fungicides)

- Get rid of the weeds (herbicides)

- Promote growth (fertilizers and hormones)

- Cut back on rot (preservatives) and infection (antibiotics)

Only a small amount of these substances get into the food, and your body can usually get rid of them pretty fast. Some can stick around a bit longer than others; some can hang out in fat tissue for a long time. Because so many of our foods are treated with these chemicals, there may be an additive effect, where we end up exposed to more than our bodies can healthily handle. Chemicals in food affect people who are actively growing more than people who are fully grown. That's because what we eat and drink become your body's building blocks. For girls who are both growing up and growing breasts, we think it's important to be extra-careful. Your newly built breasts are the foundation of your future breast health.

The fact is that we don't know a ton about the safety of various foods, beverages, and other products relative to a girl or woman's breast health, because it hasn't been carefully studied. But with what we do know today about the presence of chemicals in food, there are reasons for concern. Knowing how much is at stake—you and your health—and based on our limited understanding at this time, we want you to be thoughtful about these everyday choices so you can have the best breast health possible. The easiest ways to find healthy foods to eat, beverages to drink, and products to use is to go organic.

Many of the same breast-healthy steps are also good for the planet. Really, the outside environment and your inside environment are totally connected through the food you eat, the beverages and water you drink, the air you breathe, and more.

Eating Organic Foods and Beverages

What goes in your grocery cart is under your and your family's control. Read the labels on the food packages in order to figure out what's inside (and what's not). You want to pick products that are described by terms that mean something and avoid products with empty claims.

Words such as *organic* can be meaningful or meaningless. The United States Department of Agriculture (USDA) has specific rules about using the word *organic* to describe how food is grown and produced.

Even though a number of these terms are without an official definition and are unregulated, there are truth-in-labeling laws that say that no manufacturer can mislead the public with false claims. Great idea—but not something we can depend on.

In general, organic foods have about two-thirds fewer pesticides than nonorganic foods. That's a big difference. While terms like "natural" and "simple" might sound good, they have no official meaning. The nonprofit organization Healthy Child Healthy World has leading experts such as Dr. Harvey Karp to provide you and your family with a cleaner, greener, and safer home and food choices. See their book *Healthy Child Healthy World* and their Web site, www.healthychild.org.

The more ingredients in food, the harder it is to track down how each was made or grown and the more difficult it is to certify it as organic. When you're reaching for something to eat, try to grab something that is fresh, whole, unprocessed, grown locally, and pesticide-free and hormone-free.

what do all of the terms on food labels mean?

- 100% Organic means all product ingredients are organically grown or produced (without toxic pesticides, artificial fertilizers, synthetic hormones, antibiotics, irradiation (to kill bacteria), genetic engineering of the seeds or plants, or any sewage or sludge (in some places human poop is used as a fertilizer—*gag*).

- USDA Organic means that at least 95 percent of the product's ingredients (by weight) are organic. It's particularly important to look for this label on meats and dairy products (for more information, go to www.ams.usda.gov/nop).

- Made with organic ingredients means that at least 70 percent of the ingredients are organically grown.

- No antibiotics and Raised without antibiotics are an official definition (meaning that the food was grown or raised without antibiotics) but this food label claim is mostly unregulated.

- Pesticide-free, No pesticide residue, and Nontoxic all sound straightforward but are without official definitions and are unregulated.

- rBGH-free or rBST-free (referring to an artificially produced growth hormone given to dairy cows to increase their milk production) sounds straightforward but has no official definition and no "food police" to make sure farmers fulfill the claim.

- GMO-free means it contains no genetically modified organisms, referring to foods whose seeds were changed by putting in a new gene or modifying one that's already there.

- Grass-fed animals were raised on at least 80 percent grass or other greens in pastures or forests instead of grains.

- No hormones administered means that the beef or other farm animals have never received supplemental hormones.

- Free-range chicken or turkeys means that they are raised in a pen with room to move around, rather than cramped up in a cage packed with other birds.

- Nutriclean is a defined and regulated term meaning that fruits and vegetables have a pesticide level that's 0.05 ppm (part per million) or less.

- Natural and Simple sound good but have no official definition and are unregulated, so they mean very little.

Because organic foods tend to cost more, it makes sense to be selective with your organic choices. You want to save your money for the foods and beverages that you consume the most of and which are most likely to contain significant levels of the chemicals described above, such as apples, potatoes, peanut butter, dairy products, and beef.

Fruits and Veggies

Five to nine fruits and vegetables a day, of various colors and types (believe it or not, different-colored fruits and vegetables contain different amounts of vitamins and minerals), are important for your breast health—but only if the produce is healthy.

Fruits and veggies are most likely to contain pesticides if they are fragile, ripen quickly (chemicals may be used to slow the ripening process), have a short growing season (chemicals may be used to extend their shelf life), come from far away (they need to last longer, during transportation), and are grown in countries without laws restricting pesticide use or without enforcement of organic guidelines.

We strongly recommend eating the whole fruit or veggie whenever possible. An apple is better than a bowl of applesauce because it has more fiber and most likely less sugar. A baked potato is better than packaged mashed potatoes and french fries.

The twelve fruits and vegetables (as well as the juices that come from them) that often contain the most pesticides are peaches, strawberries, nectarines, apples, spinach, celery, pears, bell peppers, cherries, potatoes, lettuce, and imported grapes. Fruits and vegetables with relatively lower levels of pesticides include bananas, mangoes, pineapple, corn, cauliflower, broccoli, asparagus, and cabbage. These pesticide test results don't necessarily apply to all sources of each fruit. For example, some sources of bananas could have higher levels of pesticides and some grapes lower levels.

The information in the chart on the next page, on forty-three fruits and vegetables, was prepared by the nonprofit organization: Environmental Working Group (www.foodnews.org).

PESTICIDES IN: 43 FRUITS AND VEGGIES

RANK	FRUIT OR VEGGIE	SCORE
1 (worst)	Peaches	100 (highest pesticide load)
2	Apples	96
3	Sweet bell peppers	86
4	Celery	85
5	Nectarines	84
6	Strawberries	83
7	Cherries	75
8	Lettuce	69
9	Grapes, imported	68
10	Pears	65
11	Spinach	60
12	Potatoes	58
13	Carrots	57
14	Green beans	55
15	Hot peppers	53
16	Cucumbers	52
17	Raspberries	47
18	Plums	46
19	Oranges	46
20	Grapes, domestic	46
21	Cauliflower	39
22	Tangerines	38
23	Mushrooms	37
24	Cantaloupe	34
25	Lemons	31
26	Honeydew melon	31
27	Grapefruit	31
28	Winter squash	31
29	Tomatoes	30
30	Sweet potatoes	30

31	Watermelon	25
32	Blueberries	24
33	Papaya	21
34	Eggplant	19
35	Broccoli	18
36	Cabbage	17
37	Bananas	16
38	Kiwi	14
39	Asparagus	11
40	Sweet peas, frozen	11
41	Mangos	9
42	Pineapples	7
43	Sweet corn, frozen	2
44	Avocado	1
45 (best)	Onions	1 (lowest pesticide load)

Testing done on washed (e.g., apples) or peeled (e.g., bananas) fruit by the U.S. Department of Agriculture and the U.S. Food and Drug Administration.

Meat, Poultry, and Dairy

It seems like everyone's talking about issues around eating meat, poultry, and dairy products. Are they really healthy? Or are they dangerous? What's the deal?

Just as you have to watch the food you eat, you also have to watch out for what your food eats! So if you enjoy red meat, such as steak, hamburgers, salami, and hot dogs, it matters what the cows and pigs ate before they got to your plate. It is also true that if you like milk and cheese, it matters what the dairy cow ate, since the stuff in her diet goes into her milk. Here are some things you should know:

- Cows fed on grass are exposed to fewer pesticides than when they're given a diet of grain.

- Hormones given to dairy cows to increase their milk production go into their milk supply. The most commonly used dairy cow growth hormone is rBGH or rBST.

- Hormones given to beef cows to make them get bigger faster also get into their meat and fat.

- Antibiotics given to any animal to help it fight off infection can also get into its milk and meat.

- Preservatives put in processed and packaged meats, such as the nitrites in hot dogs, bacon, and bologna, are unhealthy.

- The feed given to chickens and turkeys has a big impact on the nutritional quality of their meat. The quality of the food given to hens affects the health and nutritional value of their eggs. It's best when these animals are given organic feed without pesticides and antibiotics. (Hormones are not allowed to be given to chickens or hens.)

Eating some of these foods from non-organic sources on occasion is probably harmless. But a significant amount of these products over time may prove harmful. Bottom line: it is best to avoid or reduce the amount of these chemicals in your food.

The easiest way is to buy USDA-certified organic meats and dairy products. On milk carton or bottle labels, look for the words "rBGH-free" or "rBST-free." Buy cheese that comes from organic farms or from countries that don't allow hormones to be given to dairy cows such as Canada, Australia, New Zealand, Japan, and the European Union (Holland, France, Italy, Germany, and Spain).

Limiting your consumption of red meat (beef, pork, lamb) to once or

girl to girl

I've explored cooking since I learned all this information about food. In my botany class, we studied the incredible diversity of food in the plant kingdom, so I'm also experimenting with vegan cooking. Recently, I made vegan ice cream with coconut milk and soy milk. It was so good! It's also nice knowing exactly what's going into the food I eat. If I pick my ingredients carefully, I don't have to worry about any lurking preservatives or chemicals.

twice a week will also help lower your risk of breast cancer (but these studies didn't factor in whether the red meat was organic or not. Pork and lamb are also red meat). Also, avoid grilling meat until it's black all over. And try to find lean cuts from grass-fed animals.

Whenever possible, buy meat, dairy, fruit, and vegetables from local sources. Local farms may be less likely than big companies involved in mass food production to use large amounts of harmful chemicals in the production of their food. It's also better for the environment because there is less fuel used in the transportation of the food.

Fish

In general, fish is a healthy food, but some types of fish are healthier than others. The connection between fish health and breast health is mostly unknown. Relatively high levels of polychlorinated biphenyls (PCBs), found as contaminants in big fish such as tuna, swordfish, and shark, are not breast-healthy. Mercury, also found in these big fish, has no known connection to breast health but is overall unhealthy.

There are no organic standards or rules for fish safety. Smaller fish tend to have lower levels of chemicals. The health and quality of fish depend on the water they swim in and the food they eat. One source of fish—wild (caught in their natural habitat) or farmed (raised in tanks or pens)—is not necessarily better than the other sources, but many people believe that

girl to girl

When my dad isn't working as a pediatrician in Philadelphia's Children's Hospital, he's usually fishing. I love going with him, and we catch a lot of striped bass and bluefish. Striped bass is my favorite, but we always catch more bluefish. Bluefish is a fatty fish that tends to hold on to chemicals from the water and from the smaller fish it eats, which it takes in through its gills. My family eats it no more than once or twice a week because of that. We make a really yummy bluefish pâté with the extra fish, freeze it in glass containers, and eat it later during the year once the fishing season is over.

wild fish tend to be healthier than farmed fish. This is probably true for salmon: wild salmon generally has lower levels of PCBs and mercury than farm-raised salmon. But when it comes to other types of seafood, a lot depends on what kind it is and where it comes from.

Processed Foods

The best foods are fresh, simple, whole, and organic. But most of the foods in the grocery store are processed. They are cheap, fill you up, and give you fast energy—but with little nutrition. Their list of ingredients is long and usually not organic, loaded with sweeteners, fillers, thickeners, fake color, and preservatives. Plus valuable fiber, nutrients, vitamins, and minerals are missing. Bottom line: we suggest you avoid processed foods or limit your use of them and stick to the whole good stuff.

Water

Water comes from many different places. Kitchen sink water is usually just as healthy or better than bottled water, depending on its source. Public water from your town is usually just fine, but well water may be unsafe to drink, depending on where you are, as chemicals from the ground can leach into the water. Filters can help clean home water. You can also buy distilled or purified water. To find out about the safety of your tap water, check out the Environmental Working Group's Web site: www.ewg.org/tapwater/yourwater.

The biggest issue with bottled water is the container that it comes in—usually plastic. It's both a breast health issue and an environmental concern. Even though plastic bottles are everywhere, you do have other options. TakingCareOfYourGirls.com features water bottles. Kleen Kanteen makes a stainless-steel bottle and Sigg makes an aluminum version (sold online), both metal water bottles are the ideal alternative to plastic and can be refilled with tap water. Their price tag is high ($15 to $25), but think about the money you *won't* be spending on bottled water. You'll make back your investment in no time, and you'll also make the environment *so much* happier ☺.

Plastic contains unhealthy substances that can leach out of the plastic into food or drink. One chemical is called bisphenol A, which acts a little bit like the hormone estrogen. Another is called phthalate, which also has weak hormonal activity. These chemicals are more likely to leak out when the plastic is older, has little cracks, and has been washed, heated, or frozen many times. These chemicals are also more likely to leak out into high-fat (e.g., cream soup) or acidic (e.g., tomato sauce) foods when they are stored in plastic.

Not all plastics are the same. Look at the bottom of the plastic container to see what kind of plastic it's made of—there is usually a triangle with a number between 1 and 7 in the middle. The plastic containers marked by 1, 2, 4, and 5 are believed to be safer than the ones marked 3, 6, and 7. Some plastic bottles are marked with the letters LDPE, which stands for "low-density polyethylene," a better option than PVC-containing products. But we only know a little about all of them. For sure, more studies need to be done so we can all get smarter about their safety.

The commonly used hard plastic water bottle made of polycarbonate (#7) can leach bisphenol A. Most bottled water is sold in #1 polyethylene bottles. You can refill them a few times with tap water and then recycle them.

When you're at home or at a friend's house, drink tap water from a glass. Milk and other beverages may come in #2 plastic bottles, similar to #1.

Safe Food Preparation, Utensils, and Storage

The healthiest way to cook foods is by steaming, poaching, sautéing, roasting, grilling, and microwaving (although microwaving can make your food taste weird sometimes, especially if reheating). Frying foods is unhealthy. Do your cooking and heating in pans, pots, and containers made of stainless steel, ceramic or earthenware, or glass. Use the same materials to cover the food. Avoid nonstick-coated surfaces.

Do not use plastic pans in a regular oven (such as plastic baking bags or silicone cookie sheets or muffin pans). And don't use plastic containers or wraps in the microwave oven. Take food prepackaged in plastic out of its container and heat it up in a healthy container. You can put it on a glass or ceramic plate or a non-plastic-coated paper plate, cover it with a paper towel, and put it in the microwave. Use wood cutting boards.

Remove takeout food from its plastic container and use paper or regular plates and metal silverware or chopsticks. You can also ask the restaurant if they have biodegradable containers (some are made of cornstarch or potato starch), which are safer for you and the environment.

For storage of food, use the same safe containers noted above. Stainless steel, glass (including reusable jars), and ceramic work well in the refrigerator or freezer. For food wraps, use butcher paper, wax paper, or a paper towel (and a rubber band around the outside, to secure the cover). For plastic wrap, use ones without PVC (polyvinyl chloride), such as Glad Cling Wrap, Saran with Cling Plus, or Saran Premium Wrap. Many of the options mentioned in this section are available at www.greenfeet.com.

For cold drinks, use glass cups. Whenever possible, try to buy and

girl to girl

Whenever my family finishes up food that came in a glass jar, I make sure we don't throw out the jar. I peel off the labels, wash them out, and use them for drinking. It's actually a fun break from traditional drinking glasses. I like drinking out of a big sturdy jar.

drink beverages from glass containers (most beverage cans are lined with plastic); if only plastic is available, use 1, 2, 4, or 5 coded bottles (but not all bottles are marked with a number on the bottom ☹). You know those hard clear plastic party glasses and the big red plastic cups? They are both made of #6 polystyrene—the kind to avoid.

Ceramic mugs are best for hot drinks. If you're on the go, use a stainless-steel-lined coffee cup. Styrofoam cups or plates are a no-no—they're really bad for the environment. Hot-drink paper cups are usually lined with plastic, but because they are made in many different ways and there is no product information marked on the bottom, it's hard to generalize about their safety.

Personal Products

All the different products you use to take care of your daily needs, such as shampoo, conditioner, makeup, and lotions, contain a ton of different ingredients. At this time, the quality and content of these products are so varied and unregulated that it's tough to give any firm recommendations.

Despite the Internet rumors, there is no proven connection between antiperspirants, deodorants, and breast cancer. There is a concern about the many products that contain parabens, a group of chemicals used as preservatives, because they may have weak estrogen-like activity, which could be unhealthy for your breasts. Nothing is proven so far, but it is something to keep in mind. There is also concern that lavender and tea tree oil may have hormonal effects.

For more information and to keep abreast ☺ of what's happening, check out the Environmental Working Group's reviews of the safety of personal care products on this site: www.cosmeticsdatabase.com.

Medical Ways to Keep Breasts Healthy

There are a bunch of extra things that adult women can do to keep their breasts as healthy as possible. All of these options are explained in the risk reduction and prevention sections at www.breastcancer.org.

Keep Your Breast-Healthy Lifestyle Going!

Our survey results show that girls in middle and high schools are leading relatively healthy lives: about 90 percent of girls are involved in some regular athletic activity, whether on a sports team or as part of a community program or gym. Your family makes sure you get healthy meals on a regular basis. Few of you smoke cigarettes, and most of you said you don't drink alcohol. This is very good news, particularly if you can keep this healthy lifestyle going after high school.

But after high school, with a first job or in college, many girls give up their athletic activity and increase their use of alcohol, and some even start smoking. And also look what dorm food generally is—junk food! At George Washington University, one of the most expensive colleges in the United States, the freshman food service consists of a collection of franchises: Wendy's, Baskin-Robbins, Dunkin' Donuts, and more. Not good! No wonder girls tend to gain five to twenty pounds the first year they leave home. The challenge for you will be to keep doing all the healthy things you're doing right now, including eating well, staying physically active, and staying away from unhealthy habits such as smoking and drinking alcohol.

girl to girl

Changing all these things is a lot to handle, so take it one step at a time. I'm still slowly weaning myself off junk food. But I have always loved fruits and vegetables, so that hasn't been a problem.

Any Questions?

Are there calorie savers that can make a difference?
There are a lot of practical things you can do to trim calories without stealing the fun and enjoyment you can get from food.

- Cut out sugary drinks such as sweetened iced tea, lemonade, and soda. Instead put a piece of lemon in a glass of carbonated water or try unsweetened iced tea or Honest brand tea (many fewer calories). You could even try brewing your own iced tea.

- Stick with small portions. In restaurants, order two appetizers instead of a starter and an entrée.

- When you feel the need for large portions, fill up on raw vegetables, salad, hot-air-popped popcorn (without butter), or other low-calorie items.

- Eat broiled, baked, roasted, grilled, steamed, or poached foods; avoid fried foods.

- Put salad dressing and sauces on the side. Dip your fork in the dressing or sauce, then spear the salad—you'll get enough flavor to make it taste good while saving tons of calories. (Did you know that the biggest source of fat in a woman's diet comes from salad dressing—and that fat has more calories than protein and carbohydrates?)

- Fat is an important part of our diet, in small portions and from healthy sources. Olive oil is the best oil to cook in. Butter tastes better and is healthier than margarine. Trim off the fat on meat and chicken. Avoid eating foods high in animal fat, such as bacon and sausage.

- Simple protein foods such as egg whites and chicken broth can help save on calories, satisfy hunger, and avoid cravings. You can use egg whites for omelets or just eat the whites of hard-boiled eggs. Canned or boxed organic chicken or vegetable broth is also a great option.

- Eat fruit for dessert. Peel and cut up apples, place in oven-safe bowls, bake for 45 minutes at 350°, and watch the apples turn into an absolutely delicious dessert. Put nonfat plain yogurt on top (the sugar from the apples is enough to sweeten it).

- When you're in need of a good snack, go for raw vegetables, fresh fruit, roasted nuts, or rice cakes.
- Share your ideas and watch for other girls' tips at TakingCareOfYourGirls.com.

Do artificial sweeteners increase the risk of breast cancer?
There is no proven connection between artificial sweeteners and breast cancer risk. But artificial sweeteners have no nutritional value and they keep you in the habit of craving sweets. Artificial sweeteners can con-

fuse your body's "sugar meter," leading to changes in insulin (the hormone that regulates blood sugar) levels. Over time, this kind of habit can lead to weight gain, which is not breast-healthy.

What is the fastest and most affordable way to go organic?
The higher cost of organic foods is a big problem. But with more people buying organic foods, more companies will shift to using organic foods. The result: the price will come down, and the products should become more widely available.

Look at your eating habits and preferences. Save your organic food dollars for things you eat the most of on a day-to-day basis and the foods that most often tend to be treated with pesticides or hormones (apples, potatoes, peanut butter, and dairy products). It's also a good idea to use your organic dollars for organic meat, even if you limit the amount that you eat, because meat is likely to contain more pesticides and hormones than other sources of protein. Also, keep in mind that prepared organic foods (Amy's and Cedarwood are two popular brands) add a lot of convenience but will cost more than making organic food from scratch.

Organic products don't last as long because they are without the preservatives and other things that extend shelf life. Don't pay the extra cost for a large quantity of organic food that you're going to eat very little of, as it will go bad faster and you may end up throwing most of it out.

Local sources of organic foods are also more likely to be cheaper. Joining

> ## *girl to girl*
>
> It's never too late to make meaningful changes in your life—particularly as a young person. People are capable of enormous change, adaptation, and adjustment. You'll be amazed by how many important changes you can make, especially if you get your family's cooperation.

a food co-op where your family volunteers its time can help keep costs down. Your own garden or a community garden are also great options. Recently, too, big grocery stores such as Stop & Shop have begun to offer their own in-house organic food line (Nature's Own), which is only slightly more expensive than their non-organic produce.

You can also cut back on restaurant eating and use the money you save to buy organic foods that you prepare at home.

Do I need to stop eating the foods I like?
Going organic and limiting your exposure to unhealthy things in food doesn't mean you have to change what you like to eat. For example, eating an organic apple instead of a non-organic apple can make a real difference. The taste is the same, but the organic apple will be more nutritious—and it might have a few more blemishes. The same is true for other foods. Kashi makes some delicious organic treats that you can enjoy instead of candy bars (check out snacks and treats at kashi.com).

Use this as an opportunity to try some new things. Keep your mind open to experiencing something slightly different than what you're used to. Check out a nearby organic food store and sample some snacks.

If you're really set on keeping a few not-so-healthy foods in your diet, just limit how much of them you eat. Instead of eating chocolate doughnuts twice a week, try once a month. Let it be your treat.

I don't do any of the shopping or cooking in my family, so how can I do anything about eating healthier foods?
You do have an influence on what your family puts in the shopping cart, and your family respects your intelligence and your opinions. Your point of view counts more than you realize. You are making the decisions about what you're putting in your lunch bag from home, or what you're choosing to eat in the cafeteria. And you pick your food, drinks, and snacks on the weekends, or when running off to a game or to the movie theater.

Does washing or peeling fruit or vegetables remove the pesticides?
Washing and peeling non-organic fruits and vegetables certainly helps reduce the amount of chemicals on the outside, but it doesn't entirely eliminate them.

Peeling and washing don't eliminate the chemicals that get inside fruit and vegetables. The groundwater that the plants drink can contain chemicals that washed off the outside of the plants. To clean the outside, though, you can use a vegetable wash solution from the grocery store. Or you can make your own wash: wipe or wash first with white vinegar, then rinse with water. Peeling the fruit is a good option, but you can end up throwing away valuable nutrients right under the peel. That's another reason to buy organic sources of the peelable fruits that you consume the most of, including apples and potatoes.

What's the best place to buy organic fruits and vegetables?

Farmers' markets can be a great source. In general farmers sell all of their crops locally and in season, so they don't need to use chemicals to make the produce last through the shipping process or into the next season. Plus it's planet-friendly and economical by saving gas on shipping. To find a farmers' market near you, go to www.localharvest.org and www.ams.usda.gov/farmersmarkets/map.htm.

If you can't find a farmers' market, other great choices include health food stores and supermarkets such as Whole Foods or Wild Oats.

Is it safer to become a vegetarian?

Giving up red meat and chicken doesn't guarantee a healthy diet, but it is certainly an option. Vegetarians have to be particularly careful about the quality of their fruits and vegetables because they eat much more of them than everyone else. Buying from organic sources is particularly important. Cutting out many animal sources of protein also means finding healthy plant sources to get the nutrition you need. The main sources of protein, such as dairy, soy, and beans, should be organic.

What kind of fish is healthy to buy?

Most information on fish focuses on two things: its mercury content and the environmental impact of overfishing. The nonprofit Marine Stewardship Council helps protect the world's waters from being overfished, and it also promotes responsible fish farming. What's good for the environment is usually healthy for people, so the fish-buying guide on its Web site, www.msc.org, can tell you the most environmentally friendly fish to buy near where you live.

You can share your stories and learn more
about thinking pink and living green at:

TakingCareOfYourGirls.com

Getting the Last Word

There is only one you—and that's a very big reason to celebrate. Plus, all the hard work you put into growing, supporting, understanding, and taking care of your "girls" is another big reason to celebrate.

We're not suggesting a big fancy party or a Hollywood-style celebrity bash; rather, we're talking about enjoying your strengths and interests, addressing ways you'd like to improve, developing your own personal style, building your support network of family and friends, and taking pleasure in your everyday life.

Up to this point, we've talked about a lot of different things that may sound easy but are, in fact, really hard. Each day brings its share of on and off moments, ups and downs, and little and big steps of progress. You're not alone—all of the stories that have been sprinkled throughout this book relate shared concerns, experiences, frustrations, and lessons learned from all kinds of girls of different ages. With all the tools our book provides, you're off to a great start for a lifetime of breast health and feeling good about yourself.

Knowing about breast development, breast size, breast changes, breast cancer fears, and breast health, you'll have a better idea of what to expect, and an appreciation and acceptance of how different and special each girl really is.

Even with this book, you may find that this taking-care-of-your-"girls" stuff still seems a bit mysterious. You'll keep discovering and learning a lot along the way—including big lessons such as how to deal with your own lumps and bumps, and smaller things such as figuring out your correct bra size.

Becoming a woman goes way beyond the "girls." It's about figuring out much larger questions, including who you are and who you want to be. Expect to make mistakes and have embarrassing moments along the way. That's how we live and learn.

Putting You First

Finding the strength you need to be yourself comes in large part from trying new things and doing the things you like to do. At school there are tons of classes for you to explore and become good at: math, writing, history, science, and drama, to name a few. You can also check out extracurricular activities: the debate team, community service, drama club, movies, sports, or the school newspaper. When you like what you're doing, you can get pretty good at it, have fun, and feel good.

Now you know that you don't have to be six feet tall and 120 pounds to look good in clothes, right? Dressing the body that you have with appropri-

girl to girl

I've been a peer mentor for a group of fifteen students at my school in their freshman and sophomore years. Getting to know them over these two years has been really fun, and I'm so proud to be someone they can turn to for help. My role in their lives is something I definitely take pride in. I love being with them every morning and baking for their birthdays. I recently made all of us these fun team jackets with a cool logo on it.

Of course, no one is perfect. Just try to be the best you can be; no one is saying that you have to be the best at everything! Set your own standards and let them evolve over time. Maybe you're great at playing baseball but can't hold a tune. No big deal! There are plenty of ways to figure out what you like to do, what you're good at, whom you want to spend your time with, and what you care most about without mastering every single activity you try. You're not looking to be the best in the whole wide world—you're looking to be the best you.

ate, fitted, flattering clothes that honor who you are, express your creativity and personal style, and make a strong or good impression on others is key to presenting the best you to the world. It's a skill that's going to see you through ordinary days, proms and ceremonies, get-togethers, dating, and college and job interviews.

Of course, everyone has bad days when you can get really down on yourself, focusing on the things you don't like about yourself more than the good things. Think of yourself as a whole, beautiful person, not as a collection of defective body parts. Your breasts *are* attached to your chest; your chest *is* connected to your neck and arms. Love yourself for the whole you; don't dislike yourself for a small part of the bigger picture.

Comparing Yourself to Others

There are certain points in your life where you might feel a little more uncertain—a little more vulnerable—than other times. In middle school, doesn't it seem that *everyone* is checking *everyone* else out? Who has the newest clothes? The hottest cell phone? Who got an A? Who is thin? Curvy?

So much is new and there are so many expectations! It's a lot to handle. You might worry, "How come my breasts are so small and everyone else in my family has such big ones?" Or "Why do my breasts have to be so much bigger than all the other girls'? It's not fair!"

It's just human nature to compare ourselves to others. But we can't let it stop us from really liking the body we're in. When you see a person who seems to have it all, just know she has her own set of strengths, weaknesses, and insecurities to deal with. You can always find someone who has a better, bigger, or newer something than you have—and it's easy to get wrapped up in trying to attain those things. But in doing so, it's easy to lose sight of your own strengths and potentials.

Protecting Your Breast Health

Of course, feeling good about yourself goes way deeper than great clothes, the perfect bra, or even an exciting hobby. Becoming as breast-healthy as possible is an everyday opportunity to eat the healthiest foods and drinks, exercise regularly, manage your weight, and avoid smoking and drinking alcohol. Sticking to this plan over the years will help reduce your risk of serious health problems, including breast cancer, in the future.

There's also a lot you can do to help other people stay healthy. Adopting a healthy lifestyle as a whole family makes it easier for everyone and is beneficial to all family members. If there is someone in your life who is dealing with a breast cancer diagnosis, you can help her or him with knowledge and support. Sharing your breast health and breast cancer knowledge with others is a gift and a service to your family and community. We invite you to visit www.breastcancer.org to participate in our community service program.

Asking Questions When You Need Answers

Think of someone whom you trust and can confide in. For you, it might be a mom or stepmom or older sister. For someone else, it could be a grandmother, aunt, or best friend. For sure, talking to others about uncomfortable things takes practice. The hardest part is getting the conversation started. You have to figure out what's really bothering you. Maybe you have a mix of feelings weighing you down. Perhaps you have a bunch of questions that need answers. Maybe you can't hide what you're embarrassed about—breasts are hard to conceal! It can get confusing too, because you may want two things that don't seem to go together: privacy *and* reassurance from someone else.

You may just have a short list of basic concerns: the rash under your breasts came back and your breasts hurt before your period. Or you might have one simple request: you need a new bra. No matter how big or small your questions and concerns are, they all require some form of communication.

Speaking Up for Yourself

You want to learn how to represent yourself (not have someone else speak for you) and tell your own stories. It means speaking up to your close family members and friends and sharing some of your inside feelings and concerns. You also want to learn how to share your worries with your doctor and get the answers you need on all of these sensitive topics.

In our high school surveys, girls' top two choices for whom to talk to are moms and doctors. You expect that your mom will understand; you believe that your doctor is the best source of medical information and is in the best position to reassure you. As you get close to your teens you should be able to see your doctor without your parents present. Let your doctor—and your parents—know that you'd like that privacy. This is your chance to get answers to questions and problems that may have been weighing on your mind. Unloading your worries and getting answers to your questions can make you feel much, much better. Please join us at TakingCareOfYourGirls.com to share your stories and questions.

Standing up for yourself can be incorporated into all aspects of your life. Speak up and stand up for what you believe in. Challenge what you don't agree with, support causes you believe in, and keep yourself informed.

girls call 'em ...

Air Bags
Babies
Babongas
Balloons
Bam Bams
Barbies
Bazookas
Bazooms
Ben and Jerry
Bert and Ernie
Betty and Martha
Betty Boop
Big Mamas
Bob and Fred
Bob and Joe
Bobby and Sue
Bobo and Coco
Bonnie and Clyde
Boobies
Boobillas
Booby-Woobies
Breasticles
Brita and Brenda
Bubbles
Buddies
Buddlins
Bushkas
Cha Chas
Chesticles
Coconuts
Funbags
Girlies
Goofy and Pluto
Gonzangas
Headlights
Herman and Sherman
Hooters
Humps
Jack and Jill
Jello
Jingle and Jangle
Judy and Trudy
Jugs
Knockers
Ladies

Speaking up for yourself also means speaking nicely to yourself, focusing on your strengths, and not dwelling on your weaknesses. Be kind to and take pride in yourself.

Keeping Your Self to Yourself

Your privacy is very important. You don't have to talk to people you don't want to talk to. Just because someone wants to talk to you or share secrets with you doesn't mean you have to participate. Sharing your thoughts and feelings are gifts to people around you. They are lucky to have won your friendship, your trust, and the opportunity to hear what's on your mind.

You want to be able to share what you want, keep some things to yourself, and expect people to respect your privacy. Good friends are going to understand when you set limits on how much you want to share. The better you protect their privacy, the more they'll learn the value of guarding yours.

All the confidence that comes from knowing, presenting, and speaking up for yourself will really help during the tough "teasing" years. As you learn how to handle rude or mean comments, the teasers will likely grow up a bit, deal with their own insecurities, and get a life of their own.

Reward Yourself

Each time you learn, do, share, and create good things, stop, give yourself credit, and find a way to feel good about who you are and reward what you've just accomplished. A big smile in the mirror, a pat on the back, a gift to yourself, or time off for fun can all make you feel even better about yourself. You can do this on big and small scales. After you finish a big homework assignment, let yourself finish the drawing you've been wanting to complete or indulge yourself in your favorite book for a bit. If you got that summer job you've been dying for, celebrate with some family or friends and go out to dinner.

Celebrate the people you care about by saving your energy for them. You're going to be leaning and counting on each other for good advice, good times, good stories, and all kinds of exciting things in the future.

All this knowledge is power.

You have the power to be yourself, the power to appreciate and celebrate yourself, and the power to protect and cherish your precious life. By combining your personal power with your caring and sensitivity to others, you can be ready for all the exciting things that will happen in your life. We hope that this book has been useful, informative, interesting, comforting, and good for a few laughs as you get ready for the big changes happening now and the ones to come. Put us on your shelf or under your bed and reach for us when you need to.

girl to girl

My boobs have stuck by me—well, *on* me—from the moment they started to grow. They've grown and changed as much as I have over the years, and if there's one thing I've learned from my "relationship" with my breasts, it's that they and I deserve respect, power, fun, and appreciation, from myself and everyone else. Let's face it—boobs are great. It's just learning to love what I have, no matter what, that takes the most time and patience.

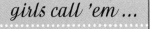

girls call 'em ...

Lady Bugs
Lady Lumps
Lilo and Stich
Lucy and Ethel
Lucy and Pierre
Mac and PC
Mammaries
Mammary Glandular Tissue
Mary-Kate and Ashley
Melons
Milk Duds
Milkshakes
Moguls
My Humps
Nuggets
Pectoral Splendor
Peter and Darcy
Princesses
Pookies
Puppies
Righty and Lefty
Romeo and Juliet
Sally and Lola
Salt and Pepper
Sisters
Snuggle Puppies
Speed Bumps
Stingrays
Tatas
The Boobular Area
The Cousins
The Girlies
The Girls
The Kids
Thunder and Lightning
Tic and Tac
Tiffany and Tonya
Tiny Tots
Tits
Titties
Titties Bitties
Water Balloons
Whooters
Yaboos
Yum Yums

Resources

Here are some terrific resources to gather more information.

Learn more, share your stories with us, check out more of Isabel's illustrations, and find out how to make your own nipple book at TakingCareOfYourGirls.com.

Bras

Guide for preteen and teen girls on issues surrounding puberty, breast development, and training bras:

www.myfirstbra.us

AA Lingerie, online store dedicated to small-busted women:

www.aalingerie.com

Lula Lu Petite Lingerie carries petite lingerie, AA and A cup bras:

www.lulalu.com

Bra Smyth, AA to H cups and everything in between:

www.brasmyth.com

Figleaves.com, bras, panties, swimsuits and full-figure lingerie:
> www.figleaves.com

Just My Size features bras of all sizes:
> www.jms.com

Breast health and breast cancer at

> www.breastcancer.org

Changing your breast size

"How to Make Your Breasts Look Bigger":
> http://ezinearticles.com/?How-to-Make-Your-Breasts-Look-
> Bigger&id=41852

American Society for Aesthetic Plastic Surgery and the American Society of Plastic Surgeons on breast implants:
> www.breastimplantsafety.org

American Society of Plastic Surgeons on breast reduction surgery:
> http://www.plasticsurgery.org/patients_consumers/links_
> resources/BRAVO-Pre-Surgery.cfm

Fashion tips for different figure types

Easy figure fixes: fashion solutions for your body type:
> http://fashion.about.com/cs/tipsadvice/a/figurefixers.htm

Discover the secrets of looking good whatever your shape:
> www.howtolookgood.com

Melange, dedicated to helping women feel and look amazing:
> http://www.melange4women.com/drforyoboty.html

Health and wellness

Healthy Child, Healthy World:
> www.healthychild.org

Teens Health, for teens looking for honest, accurate information and advice about health, relationships, and growing up:
> www.kidshealth.org and www.teenshealth.org

Stories, health information, and empowerment:
> www.girlshealth.gov

Children's Hospital Boston's Center for Young Women's Health:
> www.youngwomenshealth.org

iEmily, health and wellness site just for girls:
> www.iemily.com

Girls Inc., inspiring all girls to be strong, smart, and bold:
> www.girlsinc-online.org

For teens and young adults about health, fitness, and well-being:
> www.coolnurse.com

Online community containing stories, games, and interactive content addressing sexuality, emotions, body image, etc., for girls 13+:
> www.gurl.com

Nutrition, fitness, and weight management

Healthy Child, Healthy World:
> www.healthychild.org

Center for Young Women's Health:
> www.youngwomenshealth.org/healthyeating.html

Teen nutrition advice:

www.teennutrition.net

For teens:

http://familydoctor.org/online/famdocen/home/children/teens.html

Free nutrition, fitness, and diet information, advice, and planning (short registration required):

www.sparkteens.com

Personalized nutrition plan from USDA, to advance and promote dietary guidance:

www.mypyramid.gov

Food and Drug Administration's "How to Lose and Manage Weight":

www.fda.gov/loseweight

Making sense of healthy eating:

www.nutrition.com.sg/he/heteens.asp

Centers for Disease Control and Prevention site on bone health:

www.cdc.gov/powerfulbones

Everything you ever wanted to know about veggies, by teens for teens:

www.vegetarianteen.com

CalorieCount from About.com Health, free directory of nutrition information of many common foods:

www.calorie-count.com

Plus-size shopping

Fashion Overdose, for chic, comfy, distinctive, fun, and sensibly priced apparel:

www.fashionoverdose.com

B & Lu, plus-size fashions with unique, trend-driven styles that have a boutique feel:
> www.bandlu.com

Alight.com, plus size for full-figured women and teens:
> www.alight.com

Positive body image

Honest, accurate information and advice about health, nutrition, fitness, relationships, and growing up:
> www.kidshealth.org/teen

National Organization for Women (NOW) Love Your Body campaign:
> www.loveyourbodynowfoundation.org

Dove Campaign for Real Beauty:
> www.campaignforrealbeauty.com

Safe food selection and handling (storage, carrying, reheating, etc.)

Healthy Child, Healthy World:
> www.healthychild.org

Teens Health:
> www.kidshealth.org/teen/food_fitness

Food safety education materials for kids and teens from USDA:
> www.fsis.usda.gov/Food_Safety_Education/For_Kids_&_Teens

Safety of plastics

National Geographic's The Green Guide—*green living tips, product reviews, environmental health news:*
> www.thegreenguide.com

The Green Guide, *article on plastic water bottles. Check out "related" articles on sidebar:*

> www.thegreenguide.com/doc/101/plastic

Healthy Child, Healthy World:

> www.healthychild.org

Teasing and/or bullying

Stop Bullying Now!:

> www.stopbullyingnow.hrsa.org

STOP Cyberbullying—what it is, how it works, and how to understand and deal with cyberbullies:

> www.stopcyberbullying.org

Index

Accessories, 142–143, 144
Accessory breast, 75, 77
Acetaminophen, 89
Acid washes, 65
Acne, 58, 60–61, 63, 65–66
Age
    breast cancer and, 170,
        173–175, 180, 185
    breast size and shape
        and, 32, 36, 37
Age spots, 60
Agriculture, United States
    Department of
    (USDA), 202, 203
Alcohol use, 177, 197–198,
    213
Allergic reactions, 61
American Society for
    Aesthetic Plastic
    Surgery, 166
Anorexia, 34, 40
Antibiotics, 201
    in animal feed, 39, 203,
        207
Antifungal medications, 67
Antiperspirants, breast
    cancer and, 174, 178,
    212

Areolas
    bumps on, 74
    changes in, 46
    defined, 13
    development of, 16–18
    hair around, 73, 76–77
    Montgomery glands on,
        23, 74
    size and color of, 18,
        22–23, 54, 70, 72, 76
    uneven-sized, 33
Artificial sweeteners,
    214–215
Aspiration, 52–53
Aspirin, 89
Athletic/sports bras, 60,
    62, 89, 120, 121, 128–129
Atypical breast cells, 83, 88
Augmentation surgery
    (implants), 21, 40, 152,
    153, 158–159, 162–166,
    188

Baby powder, 61, 66
Bactroban, 74
Benzoyl peroxide, 65–66
Biopsy, 53, 55–56, 90, 91,
    181

Birth control pills, 32, 89,
    155, 178–179, 200
Birthmarks, 58, 62
Bisphenol A, 210
Blood sugar, 30
Body fat, breast size and,
    30–31, 37, 38, 40
Body hair, 38
Bottled water, 209–210
Boys, breast development
    in, 11–12, 19–21
Bras, 11, 117–135, 142
    athletic/sports bras, 60,
        62, 89, 120, 121, 128–129
    band and cup size,
        122–123, 131–133
    cami (camisole), 127
    color and pattern of, 130
    comfort, 130–131
    fabrics, 131
    falling straps, 133–134
    finding right fit, 124–126
    minimizer, 134
    molded, 128
    nighttime/sleeping bras,
        89, 135, 169, 179
    not wearing, 37
    number needed, 133

Bras *(cont'd.)*
  padded and push-up,
    128, 132, 157
  parts of, 122
  plus sizes, 134
  posture and, 147
  racer-back, 129
  resources, 227–228
  special occasion, 129–130
  strapless and
    convertible, 129, 133,
    134
  strap size, 123–124
  styles of, 126–130
  talking about, 117–120
  thin-cup, 128
  training, 118, 120, 127
  underwire, 126, 127–128,
    134
  washing, 132–133
Breast augmentation, 21,
    40, 152, 153, 158–159,
    162–166, 188
Breast buds, 13–16, 81, 88
Breast cancer, 2, 43, 45, 84,
    90, 135, 167–191
  age and, 170, 173–175,
    180, 185
  breast-feeding and, 176,
    188–189
  breast surgery and, 165,
    188
  causes of, 172–173
  deodorants/
    antiperspirants and,
    169, 174, 178, 212
  ethnic groups and,
    189–190
  family history and, 52,
    54, 170, 173, 175,
    185–186, 190–191
  genetic abnormality
    and, 172–173, 175, 185,
    186, 188
  incidence of, in teens,
    170
  mammograms and, 44,
    45, 51–52, 54, 91, 180,
    181
  myths concerning, 6,
    169, 174, 178–179, 212

nighttime bras and, 169,
    179
  personal history of, 176
  recurrence of, 176, 187,
    189
  risk factors for, 174–178,
    195, 196
  signs and symptoms of,
    179–181
  sun exposure and, 60
  talking about, 24–25,
    167–169
  tests, 181–182
  treatment of, 182–185,
    187
  worrying about, 16,
    167–169, 190
Breast changes, 43–56
  breast self-exam, 44, 45,
    46–50, 53–55
  bruises and bumps,
    86–87
  cysts, 33, 52–53, 84–86, 90
  doctor's exam, 50–51
  extra breast tissue,
    82–86
  fibroadenoma, 80, 83,
    84, 91
  fibrocystic breast
    changes, 85–86, 90–91
  fluid removal, 52–53
  menstrual cycle and, 53,
    79, 80, 84–87, 90
  new feelings, 46
  normal, 79–92
  noticing, 46
  pain, discomfort,
    sensitivity, and
    tenderness, 22, 79, 85,
    87–90
  talking about, 43–44,
    79–80
  tests for, 51–53, 54
Breast development, 5,
    9–26 *(see also* Areolas;
    Nipples)
  in boys, 11–12, 19–21
  breast break, 14–15
  breast gland tissue, 17–18
  embryonic, 12–14, 74
  emotions and, 12

in newborns, 23
  puberty and, 15, 37, 77
  speed of, 19, 21–22
  talking about, 9–12,
    23–25
Breast-feeding, 13, 19, 23,
    32, 155, 162, 164, 165
  benefits of, 165, 200
  breast cancer and, 176,
    188–189
  breast size and shape
    and, 72
  inverted nipples and, 72
Breast lift (mammopexy),
    161
Breast preservation
    therapy, 183
Breast radiologists, 55,
    91–92
Breasts, names for, 224,
    225
Breast self-exams, 44, 45,
    46–50, 53–55, 181
Breast size and shape, 2–3,
    18, 26, 27–41 *(see also*
    Breast surgery)
  age and, 32, 36, 37
  body fat and, 30–31, 37,
    38, 40
  bust enhancers, 157
  clothing and, 140–145 ,
    147
  comparing, 28–29, 35,
    148–149, 221–222
  diet and nutrition and,
    30–31, 39–40
  eating disorders and, 34,
    40–41
  exercise and, 37–38
  family genes and, 29–30,
    36, 156
  hormones and, 31
  large breasts, 34, 41
  narrow breasts, 33–34
  nutrition and, 30–31
  questions on, 35–41
  resources, 228
  sagging breasts, 37
  small breasts, 34
  talking about, 27–28
  teasing about, 95–115

temporary changes, 31–32
uneven, 32–33
weight and, 30–31, 37, 40–41, 155
Breast surgeons, 55, 56, 91–92
Breast surgery, 158–166
augmentation (implants), 40, 152, 153, 158–159, 162–166, 188, 211
breast cancer and, 165, 188
breast-feeding after, 162, 164, 165
breast lift (mammopexy), 161, 165
cost of, 165–166
emotional support and, 163
reductions, 21, 152, 153, 159–160, 163, 165–166
risks of, 162–163
for tubular breasts, 161, 166
Bruises and bumps, 64, 86–87
Bullying, 109, 110, 113, 115, 232
Bust enhancers, 157

Caffeine, 80, 89
Cami (camisole) bras, 127
Cancer (see Breast cancer)
Carbohydrates, 30
Carcinoma in situ, 171
Chafing, 62
Chemicals, in food, 39, 177, 201–202
Chemotherapy, 182, 183
Chest muscles, 37–38
Chocolate, 89
Cigarette smoking, 178, 196–197, 213
Clothing, 137–149, 220–221
accessories, 142–143, 144
breast size and, 140–142
directing attention and, 142–143
fabrics, 142–143, 144

first impressions, 144–145
flirty and sexy, 143–144, 148
layering, 143
resources, 228, 230–231
talking about, 137–139
undergarments, 142
Cocoa butter, 59
Cold and heat, breast size and, 31
Colon cancer, 175
Cooper's ligaments, 122
Cornstarch, 61, 66
Crow, Sheryl, 169
Cysts, 33, 52–53, 84–86, 90

Dairy foods, 206–207
Deodorants, breast cancer and, 169, 178, 212
Dermatologists, 50, 64–67
Diet and nutrition, 89, 193, 194
artificial sweeteners, 214–215
balancing diet, 200–201
bottled water, 209–210
breast cancer and, 177, 178
breast size and shape and, 30–31, 39–40
calorie savers, 213–214
fast food, 39, 200
fats, 30, 214
fish, 208–209, 217
food labels, 202, 203
food preparation, utensils, and storage, 211–212, 214
fruits and vegetables, 204–206
meat, poultry, and dairy, 206–208
organic food, 39, 202–204, 215–217
portion size, 214
processed foods, 30, 199, 209
resources, 229–230
vegetarians, 217
Dimmers, 131

Doctor's exam, 50–51
Dress codes, 138
Dressing (see Clothing)
Ductal hyperplasia, 83
Ducts, 14, 17, 18, 73, 81–82, 171–172

Eating disorders, breast size and, 34, 40–41
Embryonic breast development, 12–14, 74
Environmental Working Group, 204, 209, 212
Estrogen, 15, 31, 38, 81, 176, 210
Exercise, 177, 194, 199–200, 213
breast changes and, 46
breast size and shape and, 37–38
Extra breast tissue, 82–86
Extra nipples, 74–77

Falsies, 157
Family history, breast cancer and, 52, 54, 170, 173, 175, 185–186, 190–191
Fast food, 39, 200
Fats, dietary, 30, 214
Fertilizers, 39, 201
Fibroadenoma, 80, 83, 84, 91
Fibrocystic breast changes, 85–86, 90–91
First impressions, clothing and, 144–145
Fish, 208–209, 217
Food, chemicals in, 39, 177, 201–202
Food labels, 202, 203
Food preparation and storage, 211, 214
Freckles, 18, 58, 60, 62–63
Fruits, 204–206
Fungicides, 201

Genes, breast size and shape and, 29–30, 36, 156
Growth spurts, 21, 37

Gynecologists, 50
Gynecomastia, 19–20

Hair, around nipples and
    areolas, 46, 54, 69, 70,
    72, 73, 76–77
Harassment, 109, 110, 113
Healthy Child, Healthy
    World, 202
Height, 21, 36–37
Herbal products, 89
Herbicides, 201
Herceptin, 184
Hormonal therapy, 182, 183
Hormone replacement
    therapy, 155, 177, 200
Hormones, 15, 20–21, 31,
    38–40, 73, 81, 85–86,
    176–177
Hughes, Finola, 140
Hyperplasia, 83

Ibuprofen, 89
Implants, 152, 153, 158–159,
    162–166, 188
Insulin levels, 30
Internet teasing, 115
Invasive ductal breast
    cancer, 172
Inverted nipples, 18, 33, 70,
    72–73
Irregular menstrual
    periods, 38
Itchy nipples, 76

Jacob, Mary Phelps, 121
Jealousy, 114–115, 149
Journal entries, breast
    self-exam and, 54–55
Juvenile fibroadenoma, 84

Karp, Harvey, 202
Kashi, 216
Koch, Dan, 147

Lankenau Hospital, 5
Large breasts (see Breast
    size and shape)
Laser hair removal, 77
Laser therapy, 65
Lavender oil, 21, 212

Lesher, Henry S., 120
Lindahl, Lisa, 121
Liposuction, 164
Lobular breast cancer, 172
Lobular hyperplasia, 83
Lobules, 14, 17, 18, 81–82,
    171–172
Lopsided breasts, 32–33
Lumpectomy, 183
Lumps (see Breast
    changes)
Lymph nodes, 172, 180,
    182

Magnetic resonance
    imaging (MRI), 52, 54,
    91, 180, 181, 188
Mammary ridges, 12–14,
    74, 75
Mammograms, 44, 45,
    51–52, 54, 91, 180, 181
Mammopexy, 161
Marine Stewardship
    Council, 217
Massage, 184
Mastectomy, 183
Meat, 206–208
Medications
    for acne and breakouts,
        65–66
    allergic reactions to, 61
    birth control pills, 32,
        89, 155, 178–179, 200
    breast cancer, 183–185
    breast changes and, 46
    breast size and, 31
    pain, 89
    for yeast infections, 67
Meditation, 184
Menopause, 36, 155,
    176–177, 200
Menstrual cycle, 22, 31, 38,
    200
    breast cancer and, 176
    breast changes and, 53,
        79, 80, 84–87, 90
Mercury, 208, 209
Metabolism, 198, 200
Metastatic breast cancer,
    184–185
Miconazole, 64

Milk ducts, 14, 17, 18, 73,
    81–82, 171–172
Miller, Hinda, 121
Minimizer bras, 134
Molded bras, 128
Montgomery glands, 23, 74
MRI (magnetic resonance
    imaging), 52, 54, 91,
    180, 181, 188

Narrow breasts (see Breast
    size and shape)
Nature's Own, 215
Needle aspiration, 52–53,
    54
Negative feelings, 103,
    139–140
Neosporin, 74
Nettles, 61
Nicotine, 178
Nighttime/sleeping bras,
    89, 135, 169, 179
Nipple books, 2–4
Nipple fluid test, 52
Nipples, 69–77
    changes in, 46
    cold and wet and, 71, 74
    coverage of, 17, 128, 129,
        131
    defined, 13
    development of, 13–14,
        16–18, 74–75
    discharge, 46, 70, 72, 73,
        181
    extra, 74–77
    flat, 72–73
    hair around, 46, 54, 69,
        70, 72, 73, 76–77
    inverted, 18, 33, 70,
        72–73
    itchy, 76
    pain, discomfort,
        sensitivity, and
        tenderness, 79, 85,
        87–89
    protecting, 62
    size and color of, 18,
        22–23, 46, 54, 69–72
    talking about, 69–71
    uneven-sized, 33
Nizoral, 64

Nutrition (*see* Diet and nutrition)

Organic food, 39, 202–204, 215–217
Ovarian cancer, 175
Ovaries, 15

Padded bras, 128, 132, 157
Pads, bra, 132
Pain medications, 89
Parabens, 212
Partial breast treatment, 183, 188
Pasties, 129
Pectoralis major, 37
Periods (*see* Menstrual cycle)
Personal products, 212
Pesticides, 39, 177, 201–207, 216
Petals, 129
Phthalate, 210
Poison ivy, 61
Polychlorinated biphenyls (PCBs), 208, 209
Portion size, 214
Positive self-talk, 103
Posture, 145–148
Pregnancy, 32, 36, 40, 77, 155, 176, 188, 200
Preservatives, 201, 207, 212
Privacy, 224
Processed foods, 30, 199, 209
Progesterone, 15, 31, 81
Protein, 30
Puberty, breast development in, 15, 37, 77
Pubic hair, 15, 34, 69
Push-up bras, 128, 132, 157

Racer-back bras, 129
Radiation, 182, 183, 189
Rashes, 58, 61–62
Retin-A, 65

Sagging breasts (*see* Breast size and shape)
Saline implants, 159

Salmon, 209
Salty foods, 89
Scar tissue, 87
Secondhand smoke, 196–197
Second opinions, 91
Self-confidence and self-esteem, 6, 35
Self-exams, 44, 45, 46–50, 53–55, 181
Self-image, 95–115
Self-tanning solutions, 60
Selsun Blue, 64
Silicone implants, 159
Skin cancer, 179
Skin problems and changes, 43, 44, 46, 57–67
  acne and breakouts, 60–61, 63, 65–66
  birthmarks, 58, 62
  bruises and bumps, 64
  chafing, 62
  freckles, 18, 60, 62–63
  rashes, 58, 61–62
  stretch marks, 54, 57, 59, 64–65
  sunburn, 58, 60, 65
  talking about, 57–58
  yeast infections, 63–64, 66–67
Sleeping/nighttime bras, 89, 135, 169, 179
Slouching, 145–146
Small breasts (*see* Breast size and shape)
Smoking, 178, 196–197, 213
Special occasion bras, 129–130
Sports/athletic bras, 60, 62, 89, 120, 121, 128–129
Steroid creams, 60, 61, 67
Strapless and convertible bras, 129, 133, 134
Stretch marks, 54, 57, 59, 64–65
Sunbathing, 44, 57, 58, 179
Sunburn, 58, 60, 65
Sun protection factor (SPF), 65
Sunscreen, 58, 60, 65

Supernumerary nipples, 75
Surgery (*see* Breast surgery)
Sweeteners, artificial, 214–215

TakingCareOfYourGirls.com, 3, 5, 209, 214
Talc, 61, 66
Tanning salons, 60
Teasing, 95–115, 224, 232
Tea tree oils, 21, 212
Thick areas, 82, 180
Thin-cup bras, 128
Thyroid cancer, 175
Tinea versicolor, 63–64
Training bras, 17, 118, 120, 127

Ultrasound, 51, 90, 91, 180, 181, 188
Ultraviolet (UV) rays, 60
Undergarments, 142
Underwire bras, 126, 127–128, 134

Vegetables, 204–206
Vegetarians, 217
Victoria's Secret, 131
Vitamins, 89

Warner Brothers Corset Company, 121
Water and water bottles, 209–210
Weight
  breast cancer and, 177
  breast development and, 20, 21
  breast size and shape and, 30–31, 37, 40–41, 155
  metabolism and, 198
Whiteheads, 57
Whole Foods, 217
Wild Oats, 217

Yeast infections, 63–64, 66–67
Yoga, 183